Fast Fa

BMA
Fast Facts:
Chronic Obstructive
Pulmonary Disease

Third edition

M Bradley Drummond MD MHS
Associate Professor, Department of Medicine
Division of Pulmonary and Critical Care Medicine
University of North Carolina School of Medicine
Chapel Hill, North Carolina, USA

William MacNee MB CHB MD FRCP
Professor of Respiratory and Environmental Medicine
Centre for Inflammation Research
Queen's Medical Research Institute
University of Edinburgh Medical School
Edinburgh, UK

Declaration of Independence
This book is as balanced and as practical as we can make it.
Ideas for improvement are always welcome: feedback@fastfacts.com

WITHDRAWN FROM LIBRARY

BMA LIBRARY
BRITISH MEDICAL ASSOCIATION

HEALTH PRESS

BRITISH MEDICAL ASSOCIATION

1000753

Fast Facts: Chronic Obstructive Pulmonary Disease
First published 2004; second edition 2009
Third edition August 2016

Text © 2016 M Bradley Drummond, William MacNee
© 2016 in this edition Health Press Limited
Health Press Limited, Elizabeth House, Queen Street, Abingdon,
Oxford OX14 3LN, UK
Tel: +44 (0)1235 523233

Book orders can be placed by telephone or via the website.
For regional distributors or to order via the website, please go to: fastfacts.com
For telephone orders, please call +44 (0)1752 202301 (UK, Europe and Asia–
Pacific), 1 800 247 6553 (USA, toll free), or +1 419 281 1802 (Americas).

Fast Facts is a trademark of Health Press Limited.

All rights reserved. No part of this publication may be reproduced, stored in
a retrieval system, or transmitted in any form or by any means, electronic,
mechanical, photocopying, recording or otherwise, without the express permission
of the publisher.

The rights of M Bradley Drummond and William MacNee to be identified as the
authors of this work have been asserted in accordance with the Copyright, Designs
& Patents Act 1988 Sections 77 and 78.

The publisher and the authors have made every effort to ensure the accuracy of this
book, but cannot accept responsibility for any errors or omissions.

For all drugs, please consult the product labeling approved in your country for
prescribing information.

Registered names, trademarks, etc. used in this book, even when not marked as
such, are not to be considered unprotected by law.

A CIP record for this title is available from the British Library.

ISBN 978-1-908541-73-4

Drummond MB (M Bradley)
Fast Facts: Chronic Obstructive Pulmonary Disease/
M Bradley Drummond, William MacNee

Medical illustrations by Annamaria Dutto, Withernsea, UK.
Typesetting by User Design, Illustration and Typesetting, UK.
Printed in the UK with Xpedient Print.

COPD FOUNDATION
Take Action Today. Breathe Better Tomorrow.

Foreword
by the COPD Foundation

Choosing good health means finding a healthcare team whose members are skilled and knowledgeable in COPD diagnosis and management strategies. COPD susceptibility begins early in life and is not always linked to a cigarette. Here, having dispelled the myth that COPD is a smokers' disease, the authors' update on etiology describes the pathogenesis of COPD as multifactorial and complex, and includes heterogeneous susceptibility for low birth weight, childhood infections, environmental exposures and low socioeconomic status. It is critical to the early diagnosis and management of COPD that clinicians do not overlook a COPD diagnosis when symptomatic patients report a minimal or absent smoking history.

Considerable detail is given to the chapter on exacerbations, which for many patients becomes the single moment in time that marks a loss in their otherwise good quality of life. All the tools for treating and managing the acute exacerbation can be found in this handbook. It is paramount that clinicians not only treat exacerbations, but work equally hard to prevent them and that moment in time that patients remember as the changing point in their quality of health.

This *Fast Facts* title ends with a look at future trends like the advancing role of CT and MRI, improved diagnostic testing, biomarkers and the potential for lung repair. Perhaps the greatest future trend is prevention and the advancement of research to find those cures for COPD.

This is an easy-to-read handbook for clinicians, presenting the latest evidence to shape our understanding of COPD today and the available treatment options. Clinicians are busy. *Fast Facts: Chronic Obstructive Pulmonary Disease* presents the latest evidence with key references and key points at the conclusion of each chapter to highlight the take-home messages. It provides the necessary information to clinicians, fast.

The COPD Foundation's mission is to prevent and cure Chronic Obstructive Pulmonary Disease and to improve the lives of all people affected by COPD
www.copdfoundation.org

List of abbreviations

ACOS: asthma COPD overlap syndrome

AIDS: acquired immunodeficiency syndrome

BMI: body mass index

BODE index: a measure of disease severity that incorporates body mass index, obstruction, dyspnea and ability to exercise

cAMP: cyclic adenosine monophosphate

CAT: COPD assessment test

CNS: central nervous system

COPD: chronic obstructive pulmonary disease

CT: computed tomography

DLco: diffusing capacity in the lung for carbon monoxide (sometimes called TLco in the UK – transfer factor of the lung for carbon monoxide)

ECG: electrocardiography/electrocardiogram

FEV$_1$: forced expiratory volume in 1 second

FVC: forced vital capacity (the total volume of air that can be exhaled from a maximum inhalation to a maximum exhalation)

GOLD: Global initiative for chronic Obstructive Lung Disease

HIV: human immunodeficiency virus

HRCT: high-resolution computed tomography

ICS: inhaled corticosteroid

ICU: intensive care unit

IL: interleukin

Kco: carbon monoxide transfer coefficient (DLco/V$_A$)

LABA: long-acting β-agonist

LAMA: long-acting antimuscarinic agent

MRC: Medical Research Council (UK)

NHLBI: National Heart, Lung and Blood Institute (USA)

NIPPV: non-invasive intermittent positive-pressure ventilation

PaCO$_2$: partial pressure of carbon dioxide in arterial blood

PaO$_2$: partial pressure of oxygen in arterial blood

PDE4: phosphodiesterase 4

PEF: peak expiratory flow

SABA: short-acting β-agonist

SaO$_2$: percentage oxygen saturation of arterial blood

SGRQ: St George's Respiratory Questionnaire

V$_A$: ventilated alveolar volume, or accessible lung volume

VC: vital capacity

Introduction

Chronic obstructive pulmonary disease (COPD) is a heterogeneous collection of syndromes with overlapping manifestations. In the past, this has led to considerable variance in definitions, so the Global initiative for chronic Obstructive Lung Disease (GOLD) was implemented in order to provide some uniformity. GOLD defines COPD as: 'a disease state characterized by persistent airflow limitation that is usually progressive and is associated with a chronic inflammatory response in the airways and the lung to noxious particles or gases. Exacerbations and comorbidities contribute to the overall severity in individual patients'. Current guidelines recommend individualizing patient management based on clinical features.

Patients with COPD often make few complaints despite experiencing considerable disability. As a result, although the condition can easily be diagnosed, it frequently is not.

COPD is also associated with a number of comorbidities. While most are common conditions, they are seen more frequently in patients with COPD than would normally be expected. This has led to the concept that COPD has systemic effects, perhaps due to an underlying chronic inflammatory process. Often these comorbidities present major clinical problems in the individual patient for whom the recognition and treatment of COPD is key to management.

The relationship between asthma and COPD has been particularly troublesome. Defining asthma as 'reversible' led to the inference that COPD is 'irreversible' and, therefore, that there was nothing to 'reverse' with treatment. This incorrect belief has served only to exacerbate the underdiagnosis and undertreatment of COPD. Distinguishing between asthma and COPD is not only difficult, but may be impossible. Both conditions are associated with chronic airway inflammation, although the underlying chronic inflammation is very different in each disease. Moreover, both conditions can occur in the same individual and some patients with asthma may progress to COPD, even in the absence of smoking. The clinical problem, thus, is not whether a patient has asthma or COPD, but rather whether the asthma or COPD phenotype predominates.

Previous guidelines have emphasized treatment for patients who have lost 50–65% of their lung function. Current guidelines, however, recognize that early recognition and intervention can have substantial benefits for the patient. Although there is no cure for COPD, preventing deterioration of the condition, improving lung function and thus symptoms, and improving health status and functional ability are all attainable goals by encouraging smoking cessation alongside a combination of pharmacological and non-pharmacological management. Ultimately, this may decrease the healthcare costs associated with the disease (see page 125).

As well as addressing all the issues described above, we take a comprehensive look at the investigations used to assess the severity and stage of COPD, and the interventions that may reduce the risk of developing the condition. We cover all the latest pharmacological treatments and summarize current clinical guidelines from an international perspective.

COPD often necessitates hospitalization, but for much of the natural history of the disease it is usually managed in primary care. This handbook is a practical and accessible resource for all general practitioners, practice nurses, specialist nurses, junior hospital doctors, paramedics, medical students and other allied healthcare professionals involved in the diagnosis and management of COPD. It will also serve as a useful overview for researchers and specialists reading outside their subject area.

Acknowledgments. The authors wish to thank Dr Stephen I Rennard for his contribution to this edition and past editions of this title.

In chronic obstructive pulmonary disease (COPD), pathological changes occur in the central conducting airways, the peripheral airways, the lung parenchyma and the pulmonary vasculature (Figure 1.1). Current concepts suggest that inflammation induced by cigarette smoke underlies most pathological lesions associated with COPD. The inflammation damages lung structures, and individuals who are unable to repair this damage develop tissue alterations and functional compromise. Inflammation also

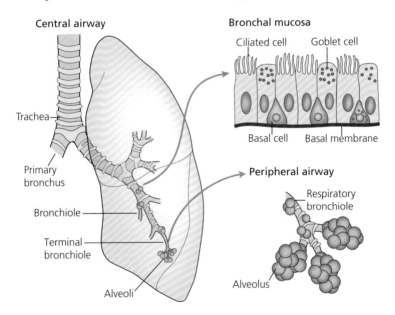

Figure 1.1 Airway anatomy: inhaled air is conducted to the alveoli through a network of bronchi (with muscular walls reinforced with cartilage) and smaller bronchioles (with incomplete muscular walls, lacking cartilage). The bronchioles connect to the alveoli. The bronchial mucosa is made of pseudostratified ciliated columnar epithelium with goblet cells and basal cells. Goblet cells have mucus granules in the cytoplasm and are responsible for secretion of mucin. Goblet cells progressively decrease in density within the peripheral airway and disappear at the level of the terminal bronchioles.

contributes to recurrent exacerbations of COPD, in which acute inflammation is superimposed on the chronic disease. There is now good evidence that all smokers develop lung inflammation; however, some individuals are more susceptible to the effects of cigarette smoke and are more severely affected.

The pathogenesis of COPD in non-smokers has not been studied as much, but inflammation secondary to air pollution or other substances is likely to play a key role. The extent of the pathological changes in the different lung compartments varies between individuals and results in the clinical and pathophysiological heterogeneity seen in patients with COPD.

Some believe that chronic asthma should be included as part of the spectrum of COPD. Although the clinical and physiological presentation of chronic asthma may be indistinguishable from that of COPD, the pathological changes are distinct from those in most COPD cases due to cigarette smoking. Histological features of COPD in the 15–20% of patients who are non-smokers have not been well studied.

Chronic bronchitis

Chronic bronchitis is defined clinically by the American Thoracic Society and the UK Medical Research Council as: 'the production of sputum on most days for at least 3 months in at least 2 consecutive years'. This chronic hypersecretion of mucus results from changes in the central airways – the trachea, bronchi and bronchioles over 2–4 mm in internal diameter. Mucus is produced by mucus glands, which are present mainly in the larger airways, and by goblet cells, found in the airway epithelium (see Figure 1.1).

In chronic bronchitis, hypertrophy of mucus glands, mainly in the larger bronchi, is associated with infiltration of the glands by inflammatory cells (Figure 1.2). In healthy never-smokers, goblet cells make up 10% of the columnar epithelial cells in the proximal airways, but their numbers decrease in more distal airways and are normally absent in the terminal or respiratory bronchioles. In smokers, however, goblet cells are not only present in increased numbers but also extend more peripherally. Metaplastic or dysplastic changes in the surface epithelium may replace the goblet cells of the normal respiratory epithelium in some smokers and thus may reduce the number of goblet cells in the proximal airways. The clinical significance of these varied anatomic alterations is unknown.

Figure 1.2 Pathological changes of the central airways in COPD. (a) A central bronchus from the lungs of a cigarette smoker with normal function shows small amounts of muscle present in the subepithelium and small epithelial glands. (b) In a patient with chronic bronchitis, the muscle appears as a thick bundle and the bronchial glands are enlarged. (c) At a higher magnification, these glands show evidence of a chronic inflammatory process involving polymorphonuclear leukocytes (arrowhead) and mononuclear cells, including plasma cells (arrow). Reproduced from the Global Initiative for Chronic Obstructive Lung Disease Workshop 2001, Original Report, with the kind permission of Professor James C Hogg, University of British Columbia, Canada.

Recent studies using bronchoscopy to obtain lavage and biopsy samples together with examination of spontaneous or induced sputum have provided new insights into the role of inflammation in COPD. Studies have reported increased numbers of neutrophils in the intraluminal space in patients with stable COPD. Bronchial biopsy studies have described inflammation in the bronchi of patients with chronic bronchitis with and without airway obstruction, and have shown that activated T lymphocytes are prominent in the proximal airways. Macrophages are also a prominent feature and, in most individuals, in contrast to asthma, the CD8 suppressor T-lymphocyte subset predominates in chronic bronchitis rather than the CD4 helper subset. Some patients with COPD, however, have a T helper cell (Th)2-type inflammation, similar to that present in asthma.

11

Neutrophils are present, particularly in the glands, in most patients with COPD, and become more prominent as the disease progresses. Nevertheless, some patients have minimal inflammation.

Bronchial biopsies taken from patients during mild exacerbations of chronic bronchitis indicate increased numbers of eosinophils in the bronchial wall, though far fewer than are present in exacerbations of asthma; increased numbers of neutrophils are also observed. Eosinophils may not be prominent in severe exacerbations. Several studies using bronchoalveolar lavage, spontaneous or induced sputum, have demonstrated intraluminal inflammation in the airspaces of patients with chronic bronchitis with or without airway obstruction. In stable chronic bronchitis, the high percentage of intraluminal neutrophils is associated with the presence of neutrophil chemotactic factors, including interleukin-8 (IL-8) and leukotriene B4, and other inflammatory mediators. There is also evidence that the airspace inflammation in patients with chronic bronchitis persists following smoking cessation if the production of sputum persists, though cough and sputum are reduced in most smokers who quit. A subset of COPD patients with eosinophils in their sputum has been described; these patients are more responsive to inhaled glucocorticoids.

Chronic inflammation of the bronchial wall is also associated with connective tissue changes that include increased amounts of smooth muscle and degenerative changes in the airway cartilage as well as increased vascularity.

Small-airways disease/bronchiolitis

The smaller bronchi and bronchioles less than 2 mm in diameter are a major site of airway obstruction in COPD. Inflammation in the small airways is one of the earliest changes in asymptomatic cigarette smokers, and considerable changes in these airways can occur without giving rise to symptoms or alteration in spirometry measurements. Thus, this region in the lung has been referred to as the 'silent zone', as abnormalities are not easily detected by conventional pulmonary function testing. The pattern of inflammatory cell changes in the small airways resembles that in the larger airways, including a predominance of CD8+ lymphocytes and an increase in the CD8:CD4 ratio.

The mechanisms leading to the increase in peripheral airway resistance include several distinct processes: destruction of alveolar support, loss of elastic recoil in the parenchyma that contributes to this support and provides driving pressure for alveolar emptying, and structural narrowing of the airway lumen. The lumen may be occluded by mucus and cells. Mucosal ulceration, goblet cell hyperplasia and squamous cell metaplasia may be present in addition to fibrosis and mesenchymal cell accumulation. As the condition progresses, structural remodeling may occur, characterized by increased collagen content and formation of scar tissue, which narrows the airways and produces fixed airway obstruction (Figure 1.3). With severe disease, the number of small airways is reduced.

Figure 1.3 Histological sections of peripheral airways. (a) Section from a cigarette smoker with normal lung function showing a nearly normal airway. (b) Section from a patient with small-airways disease showing inflammatory exudate in the wall and lumen of the airway. (c) Section showing more advanced small-airways disease with reduced lumen, structural reorganization of the airway wall, increased smooth muscle and deposition of peribronchiolar connective tissue. Images reproduced with the kind permission of Professor James C Hogg, University of British Columbia, Canada.

Pulmonary emphysema

Pulmonary emphysema is defined in structural and pathological terms as 'abnormal permanent enlargement of airspaces distal to the terminal bronchioles accompanied by destruction of their walls'. Pulmonary emphysema can also be detected radiographically, as discussed in Chapter 5. The terms used to describe emphysema are based on the anatomy of the normal lung, where a secondary lobule is defined as that part of the lung that contains several terminal bronchioles surrounded by connective tissue septa. An acinus is that part of the lung parenchyma supplied by a single terminal bronchiole. Therefore, each secondary lobule contains several terminal bronchioles and thus several acini.

Emphysema is classified by the pattern of the enlarged airspaces on the cut surface of the fixed inflated lung (Figure 1.4). Airspace enlargement can be identified macroscopically when the size of the airspace reaches 1 mm.

Figure 1.4 (a) Paper-mounted whole lung section of a normal lung. (b) Paper-mounted whole lung section from a lung with severe centrilobular emphysema; note that the centrilobular form is more extensive in the upper regions of the lung. (c) Histological section of a normal small airway and surrounding alveoli connecting with attached alveolar walls. (d) Histological section showing emphysema with enlarged alveolar spaces, loss of alveolar wall and attachments, and collapsed airways.

Absence of obvious fibrosis is a prerequisite in most definitions of emphysema; histologically, however, fibrosis has been recognized in the region of the terminal or respiratory bronchioles as part of a respiratory bronchiolitis that occurs in smokers, and lung collagen content is increased in mild emphysema.

Three principal types of emphysema are recognized according to the distribution of the enlarged airspaces within the acinar unit (Figure 1.5): centriacinar (centrilobular), panacinar (panlobular) and periacinar (paraseptal). Other, less common forms may also occur.

Centriacinar and panacinar emphysema can occur alone or in combination. Whether the two types represent different disease processes and thus have different etiologies, or whether panacinar emphysema is a progression from centriacinar emphysema is still subject to debate. The association with cigarette smoking is certainly clearer for centriacinar than panacinar emphysema, though smokers can develop both types. Those with centriacinar emphysema appear to have more abnormalities in their small airways than those with predominantly panacinar emphysema.

Centriacinar emphysema is characterized by initial clustering of the enlarged airspaces around the terminal bronchiole. It is more prominent in the upper zones of the upper and lower lobes and is the type most commonly seen in smokers.

Panacinar emphysema. The enlarged airspaces are distributed throughout the acinar unit. The destruction of the acinus is more uniform, and all of the acini within the secondary lobule are involved. In contrast to centriacinar emphysema, panacinar emphysema appears to be more severe in the lower lobe, but can be found anywhere in the lungs. It is associated with α1-proteinase inhibitor deficiency, but it can also be found in cases where no clear-cut genetic abnormality has been identified.

Periacinar (paraseptal or distal acinar) emphysema is the least common of the three main types. It is characterized by enlargement of the airspaces along the edge of the acinar unit, but only where it abuts a fixed structure, such as the pleura or a vessel. Periacinar emphysema is now a recognized emphysema pattern in smokers. It can be associated with pneumothorax.

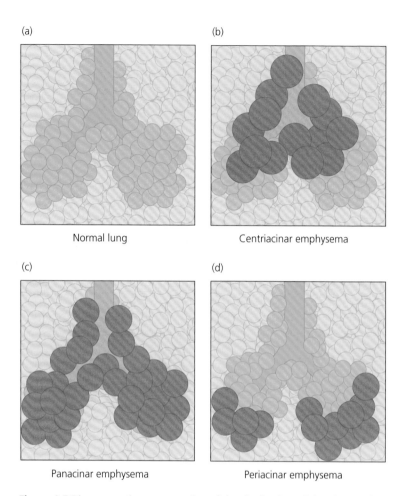

(a)

Normal lung

(b)

Centriacinar emphysema

(c)

Panacinar emphysema

(d)

Periacinar emphysema

Figure 1.5 Diagrammatic representation of the distribution of the abnormal airspaces within the acinar unit in the three major types of emphysema. (a) Acinar unit in a normal lung (although the illustration shows a clearly defined area for the purposes of clarity, it must be remembered that adjacent acinar units intercommunicate and are not necessarily demarcated by septa). (b) Centriacinar (centrilobular) emphysema: focal enlargement of the airspaces around the respiratory bronchiole. (c) Panacinar (panlobular) emphysema: confluent even involvement of the acinar unit. (d) Periacinar (paraseptal) emphysema: peripherally distributed enlarged airspaces where the acinar unit abuts a fixed structure, such as the pleura.

Unilateral emphysema or Swyer–James–MacLeod syndrome (unilateral hyperlucent lung syndrome) is a complication of severe childhood infections with rubella or adenovirus.

Congenital lobular emphysema is a developmental abnormality affecting newborn children.

Scar or irregular emphysema comprises enlarged airspaces around the margins of a scar unrelated to the structure of the acinus.

Combined pulmonary fibrosis and emphysema syndrome (CPFE) occurs when centrilobular and/or paraseptal emphysema in upper lung zones is present along with pulmonary fibrosis in lower lung zones. The physiological correlates of CPFE include unexpectedly reduced lung volumes along with frequent abnormalities in the diffusing capacity of the lung for CO_2 (DLco) and pulmonary hypertension.

Bullae are localized areas of emphysema that are overdistended. Conventionally, only lesions over 1 cm in size are described as bullae. Bullae arise in areas of lung that have been locally destroyed, though this destruction does not have to be a result of emphysema; the damage can also result from lytic or traumatic causes. They have been described in patients with tuberculosis, sarcoidosis, AIDS and trauma. The origins of bullae remain obscure. In around 20% of cases the surrounding lung is normal, but most bullae are associated with more generalized emphysema and chronic airway obstruction.

Pulmonary vasculature

The vasculature of the lung may be affected in several ways. The development of chronic alveolar hypoxia in patients with COPD results in hypoxic vasoconstriction of the small pulmonary arteries and, consequently, an inflammatory response in the arteries similar to that in the lungs. This leads to remodeling of the pulmonary arteries. As a result, early in COPD the intima may become thickened, followed by an increase in the amount of smooth muscle and infiltration of the vessel wall with inflammatory cells. As the disease progresses, the amounts of smooth muscle, proteoglycans and collagen present in the vessel wall increase and cause it to thicken. Right ventricular hypertrophy and pulmonary hypertension are common in patients with advanced COPD who have chronic hypoxemia.

Functional compromise of the pulmonary circulation can also be caused by dynamic hyperinflation, which increases intrathoracic pressure, restricts blood flow and may contribute to impaired diastolic filling of the heart.

Physiological significance

The pathological changes in patients with COPD are complex and may occur to varying extents in the large and small airways, and in the alveolar compartment. It is difficult to determine clinically or by respiratory function tests the relative contributions made to airway obstruction by the different pathological changes. In general, it is thought that the smaller bronchi and bronchioles less than 2 mm in diameter are the major sites of airway obstruction in COPD. Symptoms and physiological abnormalities in a given individual may be due to different combinations of lesions at different stages.

Narrowing of small airways can result from the formation of peribronchiolar scars and consequent contraction. Consistent with this, decreased airway circumference correlates well with airflow limitation, as does reduced numbers of small airways in patients with moderately severe COPD when assessed on specimens removed surgically.

Emphysema leads to decreased expiratory airflow by different mechanisms.

Loss of elastic recoil of the lungs, due to loss of alveolar attachments to the smaller airways, decreases the driving pressure that empties the alveoli and reduces the intraluminal pressure within the terminal airways. Because of this and because of destruction of alveolar attachments that tether the small airways in an open position, small airways can collapse during forced exhalation, resulting in effort-independent limitation of expiratory airflow.

Hyperinflation. Narrowing of the peripheral airways and the loss of elastic recoil of the lungs can also progressively trap gas during expiration, leading to hyperinflation of the lungs with over-distension of alveoli, which may also lead to airway compression. Hyperinflation reduces the inspiratory capacity so that the functional residual capacity increases, particularly during exercise. This dynamic hyperinflation is the main cause of breathlessness on exertion that reduces exercise capacity.

Intraluminal accumulation of secretions and cells may also play a role in airflow limitation.

Gas exchange abnormalities develop as the pathological changes progress, producing hypoxemia and, in some cases, hypercapnia.

Enhanced inflammatory response. The normal inflammatory response in the lungs to the inhalation of irritants, such as cigarette smoke, appears to be enhanced and abnormally persistent in patients with COPD. The factors responsible for the amplification of inflammation in COPD are not fully understood, but may involve genetic and epigenetic mechanisms. Oxidative stress, caused by an excess of oxidants in relation to antioxidants, is due to oxidants inhaled in cigarette smoke, though the release of oxidants from inflammatory cells may also enhance the inflammatory response through the activation of inflammatory genes. Oxidants also inactivate protective antiproteases and cause mucus hypersecretion.

Breakdown of connective tissue. There is good evidence that an imbalance between protease release and antiproteases in the lungs of patients with COPD leads to the breakdown of connective tissue components in the lung parenchyma, resulting in the tissue destruction seen in emphysema.

Altered structural cell function. Structural cells obtained from the lungs of patients with COPD have been shown to manifest persistently altered functions when cultured in vitro, perhaps as a result of epigenetic modifications. Lung cells have increased sensitivity to apoptosis, mediate repair functions less well and produce increased amounts of inflammatory mediators. The altered function of structural cells may account for the persistence of inflammation and progression of COPD, once established, even if cigarette smoking is stopped.

Key points – pathology and pathogenesis

- COPD results from pathological changes in the large and small airways (bronchiolitis) and in the alveolar space (emphysema).
- Chronic bronchitis is defined clinically as the production of sputum on most days for at least 3 months a year over at least 2 consecutive years.
- Inflammation occurs in large and small airways, and in the alveolar space, most commonly involving a number of cells including neutrophils, macrophages and T lymphocytes, particularly CD8+ lymphocytes.
- Small-airways disease or bronchiolitis can result in inflammation and eventually scarring of the small airways; this is an important pathological change in COPD, which is difficult to assess by respiratory function tests, but may be a major source of airway obstruction.
- Centriacinar (centrilobular) emphysema is the most common form of emphysema, particularly in smokers, and is distributed mainly in the upper zones of the lungs. Panacinar (panlobular) emphysema has a more diffuse distribution, predominantly in the lower zones of the lungs, and is associated with α1-antitrypsin deficiency; it can also occur in some smokers.
- Bullae are emphysematous spaces over 1 cm in diameter.
- Combinations of these pathological changes to varying degrees in different individuals with COPD contribute to the airflow limitation.
- The lungs of patients with COPD show an amplified and persistent inflammatory response to the inhalation of particles and gases, particularly those in cigarette smoke. A protease:antiprotease and oxidant:antioxidant imbalance is part of this amplified inflammatory response.
- Once COPD is established, the inflammatory process persists even after smoking cessation.

Key references

Barnes PJ, Shapiro SD, Pauwels RA. Chronic obstructive pulmonary disease: molecular and cellular mechanisms. *Eur Respir J* 2003;22:672–88.

Chung KF, Adcock IM. Multifaceted mechanisms in COPD: inflammation, immunity, and tissue repair and destruction. *Eur Respir J* 2008;31:1334–56.

Cosio G, Saetta M, Agusti A. Immunologic aspects of chronic obstructive pulmonary disease. *N Engl J Med* 2009;360:2445–54.

Di Stefano A, Caramori G, Ricciardolo FL et al. Cellular and molecular mechanisms in chronic obstructive pulmonary disease: an overview. *Clin Exp Allergy* 2004;34:1156–67.

Global Initiative for Chronic Obstructive Lung Disease (GOLD). Pathogenesis, pathology, and pathophysiology. In: *Global Strategy for the Diagnosis, Management, and Prevention of COPD*. Updated January 2015. www.goldcopd.org/uploads/users/files/GOLD_Report_2015.pdf, last accessed 19 January 2016.

Hogg JC. The pathophysiology of airflow limitation in chronic obstructive pulmonary disease. *Lancet* 2004;364:709–21.

Hogg JC, Chu F, Utokaparch S et al. The nature of small airway obstruction in chronic obstructive pulmonary disease. *N Engl J Med* 2004;350:2645–53.

Hogg JC, Timens W. The pathology of chronic obstructive pulmonary disease. *Ann Rev Pathol Mech Dis* 2009;4:435–59.

MacNee W. The pathogenesis of chronic obstructive pulmonary disease. *Clin Chest Med* 2007;28:479–513.

McDonough, JE, Yuan R, Suzuki M et al. Small-airway obstruction and emphysema in chronic obstructive pulmonary disease. *N Engl J Med* 2011;365:1567–75.

Saetta M, Turato G, Maestrelli P et al. Cellular and structural bases of chronic obstructive pulmonary disease. *Am J Respir Crit Care Med* 2001;163:1304–9.

Saetta M, Turato G, Timens W, Geffery P. Pathology of chronic obstructive pulmonary disease. *Eur Respir Mon* 2006;38;159–76.

Shapiro SD, Reilly Jr JJ, Rennard SI. Chronic bronchitis and emphysema. In: Mason RJ, Broadus VC, Martin TR et al., eds. *Murray & Nadel's Textbook of Respiratory Medicine*, 5th edn. Philadelphia: Elsevier, 2010: 919–67.

Voelkel NF, MacNee W, eds. *Chronic Obstructive Lung Diseases*, 2nd edn. McGraw-Hill Medical, 2009.

Washko GR, Hunninghake GM, Fernandez IE et al. Lung volumes and emphysema in smokers with interstitial lung abnormalities. *N Engl J Med* 2011;10:364:897–906.

21

The measure most commonly used to monitor the natural history of COPD is the forced expiratory volume in 1 second (FEV_1). This parameter can be readily measured by spirometry (see Chapter 4), and is justly regarded as the single most important objective measure of COPD for both research and clinical purposes. However, several other clinical parameters independently characterize the features of the disease (see Chapter 4); these clinical features do not always relate closely to FEV_1, and for this reason FEV_1 cannot be used as the sole measure of COPD severity.

Airway development and lung function

The conducting airways are fully developed by 16 weeks' gestation. Alveolar structures develop both pre- and postnatally, increasing in number in early childhood up to about the age of 8 years. Alveolar size continues to increase with lung growth.

Maximal lung function is reached in young adulthood and correlates with the attainment of maximal body size. Women achieve maximal lung function sooner than men due to their earlier growth spurt and epiphyseal closures.

Lung function, after reaching a maximum in young adulthood, remains stable for a decade or so and then begins to decline at a slowly increasing rate. On average, FEV_1 declines by about 20 mL/year after the age of 30, and by up to 30 mL/year by 70 years of age.

Risk factors

COPD has not always elicited sympathetic interest from the medical community. In their groundbreaking monograph on the natural history of COPD, Fletcher and colleagues chose the following quote to emphasize the self-perpetuating attitude that has inhibited the understanding and management of COPD.

'...medicine has come a long way since 1925, when Williams, writing Middle Age and Old Age, could confidently assert: "Chronic bronchitis with its accompanying emphysema is a disease on which a good deal of wholly unmerited sympathy is frequently wasted. It is a disease of the gluttonous, bibulous, otiose and obese and represents a well-deserved nemesis for these unlovely indulgences ... the majority of cases are undoubtedly due to surfeit and self-indulgence."'

Fortunately, great gains have been made in understanding the pathogenesis, physiology, clinical features and management of COPD. While cigarette smoking, itself now regarded as a disease, is the major risk factor, COPD also occurs in non-smokers and individuals vary greatly in their susceptibility to smoke.

Cigarette smoking is the most important etiologic factor for the development of COPD. There is a highly significant dose and duration effect, with smokers having lower lung function the more and longer they smoke. There is, however, considerable individual variation. Some non-smokers, for example, have impaired lung function. Approximately 20% of patients with COPD are lifelong non-smokers. Conversely, some heavy smokers are able to maintain normal lung function (Figure 2.1).

It is likely that smoking contributes to the development of COPD in several distinct ways and at several different periods over the lifespan of the individual (Table 2.1). Furthermore, the adverse effects of smoking on lung function are likely to be greater the earlier an individual is exposed.

Exposure to other substances, including indoor and outdoor pollution, can also contribute to the development of COPD. Passive exposure to cigarette smoke is an important risk factor and may contribute to the development of COPD in non-smokers. Individuals exposed to dusts and fumes who also smoke cigarettes have the highest risk of developing COPD.

Mechanisms of effect. The mechanisms by which cigarette smoke leads to COPD are under intensive study, as they offer potential opportunities for therapeutic intervention. Smoke is capable of inducing an inflammatory response through a number of mechanisms. It induces release of proinflammatory mediators from epithelial cells present in the lower respiratory tract, as well as from resident macrophages. It can also

23

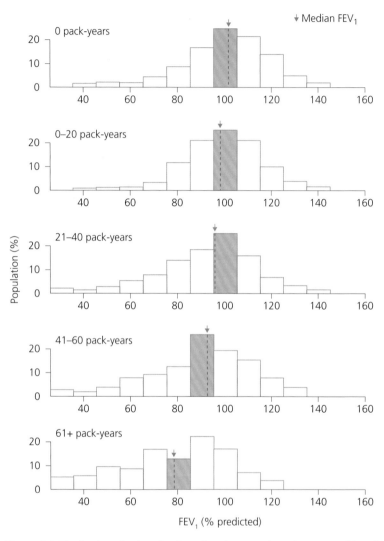

Figure 2.1 Distribution of values for forced expiratory volume in 1 second (FEV_1) expressed as a percentage of the predicted value for groups with differing smoking histories. Data from Burrows et al. 1979.

activate complement. Thus, the inflammation that is characteristically present in the lungs of smokers probably results from activation of multiple pathways. The mediators released by inflammatory cells and parenchymal cells recruited and stimulated by cigarette smoke are capable

TABLE 2.1

Mechanisms by which smoking may contribute to COPD

Prenatal exposure
- Reduced lung development
- Low birth weight

Childhood
- Decreased lung growth and thus decreased maximal attained lung function

Adulthood
- Reduction in the 'plateau phase' during which lung function remains stable in young adulthood
- Accelerated onset of lung function decline
- Lung destruction
- Impaired lung repair

of inducing lung damage. These mediators include reactive oxygen species, active proteinases and toxic peptides. In addition, cigarette smoke can decrease levels of antioxidants and antiproteinases that serve to mitigate damage caused by these toxic moieties. These effects therefore tip the balance in the lung toward tissue damage both by increasing the production of toxic mediators and by decreasing defenses.

Smoke may also alter the ability of the lungs to self-repair. This feature may resemble the widely recognized systemic adverse effect smoke has on wound healing. In other words, smoke can both increase tissue damage and impair the ability to repair that damage.

Heterogeneous susceptibility. The complex interactions between cigarette smoke and the lungs of smokers suggest multiple steps at which individual susceptibility may vary. Consistent with this, smokers show considerable heterogeneity in their susceptibility to developing COPD and strong genetic components appear to be present. Both smoking and non-smoking siblings of individuals with established COPD are at greatly increased risk of lower lung function than are siblings of individuals without COPD. It is likely that a number of specific genetic factors will affect susceptibility to COPD (see pages 27–9).

Other environmental exposures such as occupational exposures to organic and inorganic dusts, chemical agents and fumes are risk factors for COPD. Such occupational exposures contribute to 10–20% of the symptom or functional impairment in COPD. Exposure to smoke from the burning of biomass fuel for cooking or heating in poorly ventilated dwellings is an important risk factor for COPD in parts of the world where this practice is common. Exposure to high levels of urban air pollution is also a risk factor for COPD, although the level of increased risk is small compared to that of tobacco smoking.

Low maximal attained lung function increases the risk of excessive loss of lung function in later life. Not surprisingly, a variety of early life events can increase the risk for the development of COPD, presumably by affecting lung growth and development.

Low birth weight. Individuals with low birth weight, for example, have been shown to have both a reduced maximal attained lung function in young adult life and reduced lung function as they get older.

Infection. Some childhood infections have been reported both to reduce lung function in adulthood and to increase the risk of pulmonary symptoms. Interestingly, these infections may affect lung function in several ways. In addition to acutely altering lung growth and development, some infections may have direct effects in later life. Specifically, small portions of some viral genomes can be chronically incorporated and expressed in lung cells. Such expression may predispose individuals to inflammation and lung damage in later life. The lower respiratory tract, contrary to what was believed for many years, is not sterile but contains a microbiome of its own. Whether alterations in the lung microbiome play a role in COPD pathogenesis is currently under investigation.

Low socioeconomic status is also a risk factor for the development of COPD and may reflect the association with risk factors such as smoking, occupational exposures and respiratory infections.

Airway hyperreactivity is also a risk factor for the development of COPD. It is measured by challenging individuals with low doses of either the acetylcholine analog methacholine or histamine. The challenge results in constriction of airway smooth muscle and a reduction in airflow, usually measured by FEV_1. A lower dose of methacholine is required to reduce airflow by 20% in hyperreactive airways than in normal airways (Figure 2.2). The fact that asthma is characterized by increased airway reactivity and individuals with increased reactivity have a greater risk of developing COPD suggests a link between asthma and COPD. Consistent with this, a proportion of patients with asthma appear to have an accelerated rate of decline in lung function suggestive of COPD.

Chronic bronchitis or mucus hypersecretion is associated with increased FEV_1 decline; younger adult smokers with chronic bronchitis have an increased risk of COPD.

Genetic factors. There is a significant familial risk of airflow limitation in smoking siblings of patients with severe COPD, suggesting that genetic

Figure 2.2 Airflow in hyperreactive airways is reduced by a lower dose of methacholine than airflow in normal airways. Here, the normal and asthmatic responses to a methacholine challenge are plotted in terms of the forced expiratory volume in 1 second (FEV_1), expressed as a percentage of the baseline value, against methacholine dose. A significant reaction is defined as a 20% drop in FEV_1. The dose at which this occurs is termed the PD_{20}. The lower the PD_{20}, the more reactive the airways.

factors influence the development of the condition (Table 2.2). The most widely recognized genetic association with COPD is α1-proteinase inhibitor deficiency (α1-antitrypsin deficiency). About 1 in 2500 individuals in the USA has a severe deficiency, which may account for about 2% of all patients with emphysema. People deficient in α1-proteinase inhibitor are at increased risk of developing COPD even if they do not smoke, although not all affected individuals develop disease. If such individuals smoke, they are much more likely to develop severe COPD and to develop it at a particularly early age (Figure 2.3).

α1-proteinase inhibitor is a major inhibitor of serine proteinases, including neutrophil elastase; thus, it is postulated that α1-proteinase inhibitor deficiency results in excess activity of neutrophil elastase and therefore tissue destruction and emphysema. However, only some non-smokers with α1-proteinase inhibitor deficiency develop emphysema. Some maintain normal lung function throughout life. This indicates the importance of other factors.

TABLE 2.2

Components possibly related to genetic pathogenesis of COPD

- α_1-proteinase inhibitor
- α_1-antichymotrypsin
- α_2-macroglobulin
- Serine protease inhibitor nexin 2
- Matrix metalloproteinase-1
- Matrix metalloproteinase-9
- Matrix metalloproteinase-12
- Microsomal epoxide hydrolase
- Glutathione S transferase
- Heme oxygenase 1
- Cytochrome P450 1A1
- Vitamin D-binding protein
- Tumor necrosis factor α
- Interleukin-1

- Interleukin-1 receptor antagonist
- Interleukin-11
- Transforming growth factor β1
- Transforming growth factor β receptor 3
- Transforming growth factor β2
- Cystic fibrosis transmembrane regulator
- α_2-adrenergic receptor
- ABO-secretor status
- Microsatellite instability
- Hedgehog interacting protein
- FAM13A
- RIN3
- Nicotinic receptor α3

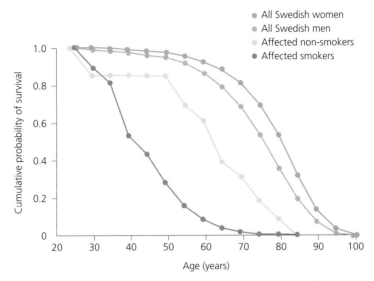

Figure 2.3 Cumulative probability of survival after 20 years of age for smoking and non-smoking individuals with α1-proteinase inhibitor deficiency compared with the total population. Data from Larsson 1978.

Additional genetic associations that may contribute to COPD risk and that are more common than α1-proteinase inhibitor deficiency have been identified, although these are likely to increase the risk of COPD only modestly. Interestingly, many of these candidate genes can affect proteinase or oxidant balance, suggesting mechanisms of action analogous to those in α1-proteinase inhibitor deficiency.

Inhibition of tissue repair may contribute to the development of COPD alongside the mechanisms that augment tissue destruction. Starvation, for example, has been reported to cause COPD both in humans and in animals. Moreover, starvation can exacerbate proteinase-induced emphysema in animal models. Such a mechanism may have clinical relevance. Many individuals with seemingly stable COPD often deteriorate if they develop a severe and prolonged intercurrent illness. Thus, one of the benefits of careful attention to nutritional balance in such patients might be mitigation of the acceleration of COPD.

Other factors can also contribute. For example, emphysema has been reported in patients with HIV infection. In this context, the inflammation

29

associated with HIV may be a contributing factor independent of cigarette smoke.

Progression of clinical symptoms

Current understanding of the natural history of COPD depends on assessment of FEV_1. However, there is considerable heterogeneity in FEV_1 decline in observational cohort studies. The ECLIPSE study, a 3-year observational study of 2164 individuals with COPD, observed that 38% of participants had an estimated FEV_1 decline of more than 40 mL/year, 31% declined by 21–40 mL, while 23% had a change ranging from 20 mL/year loss to 20 mL/year increase. This heterogeneity in FEV_1 decline highlights the importance of assessing other clinical disease parameters in COPD independent of FEV_1.

The COPD Foundation Guide to COPD Diagnosis and Treatment (see Useful resources) recommends assessment of seven severity domains, each of which can affect therapeutic approaches: airflow (FEV_1), symptoms, presence of exacerbations, oxygenation, emphysema, chronic bronchitis, and presence of comorbidities. Weight loss, for example, is a bad prognostic sign; survival in patients with COPD is negatively correlated with body mass index (Figure 2.4). Similarly, measures of health status (or 'quality of life') correlate significantly, but weakly, with FEV_1. Other factors such as exacerbations seem to be more important in driving health status, particularly in severely affected individuals.

It is important, therefore, to view the natural history of COPD not only in terms of the decline in FEV_1, but also in terms of increasing symptoms. Figure 2.5 indicates the average age of onset of symptoms. Many individuals will have symptoms at a much earlier stage, and some will progress to very limited airflow without being symptomatic. Cough and sputum production, the defining features of chronic bronchitis, can be present independently of airflow limitation.

In addition, dyspnea is not directly related to FEV_1. Rather, with exertion, tachypnea ensues. This can lead to dynamic hyperinflation, and it is the increase in inspiratory work caused by hyperinflation that is generally perceived as dyspnea. Many people who are developing COPD control dyspnea on exertion by decreasing their level of effort. As a result, they forgo activities as their disease progresses. Often this is attributed to

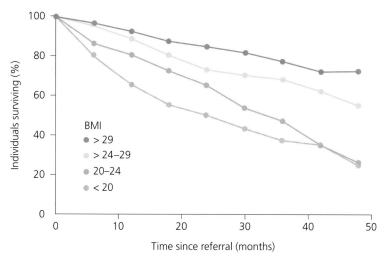

Figure 2.4 Weight as a prognostic sign in COPD: survival is negatively correlated with body mass index. The data represent 400 consecutive patients with COPD referred for rehabilitation, who received no special dietary intervention. BMI, body mass index (mass [kg]/height^2 [m^2]). Data from Schols et al., 1998.

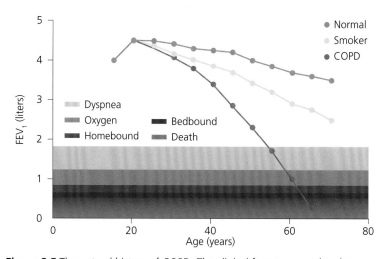

Figure 2.5 The natural history of COPD. The clinical features are related to averages for forced expiratory volume in 1 second (FEV$_1$); there are marked individual variations. Data adapted from Fletcher et al. 1976, 1977. Recent data suggest that lung function loss may slow as the disease becomes more severe.

aging or is accepted as 'normal' in a smoker, and subjects can become severely limited before presenting with symptoms.

The fact that individuals with COPD can have physiological limitation and restricted activity at early stages of the disease without complaining of symptoms is a major reason for encouraging early diagnosis, which requires spirometry. Initiation of appropriate therapy early may improve patient function and quality of life, while preventing the severe deconditioning that routinely accompanies progressive COPD. Early recognition and intervention is a major goal of current recommendations, including those of the Global initiative for chronic Obstructive Lung Disease (GOLD), the American Thoracic Society/European Respiratory Society and the COPD Foundation, and contrasts with older staging systems, in which a greater emphasis was placed on end-stage disease.

Key points – etiology and natural history

- Cigarette smoking is the most important risk factor for COPD; about 80% of patients with COPD are, or have been, smokers.
- Almost all smokers develop impaired lung function.
- Other influences, including air pollution and occupational exposures, contribute to COPD risk.
- Individual genetic susceptibility probably accounts for the heterogeneity of COPD risk.
- It is likely that many specific genetic factors will contribute to COPD risk; α1-proteinase inhibitor deficiency is the best characterized of these.
- Asthma may contribute to COPD risk in some individuals.
- Early life events, including compromised lung development and growth, are likely to contribute to the risk of developing COPD later.
- Many individuals with COPD are undiagnosed, as symptoms of dyspnea can be minimized by restricting activity, which leads patients to discount their functional compromise.

Key references

Barker DJ, Godfrey KM, Fall C et al. Relation of birth weight and childhood respiratory infection to adult lung function and death from chronic obstructive airways disease. *BMJ* 1991;303:671–5.

Burrows B, Knudson RJ, Cline MG et al. Quantitative relationships between cigarette smoking and ventilatory function. *Am Rev Respir Dis* 1979;115:751–60.

Fletcher C, Peto R. The natural history of chronic airflow obstruction. *BMJ* 1977;1:1645–8.

Fletcher C, Peto R, Tinker C, Speizer FE. *The Natural History of Chronic Bronchitis and Emphysema: An Eight-Year Study of Early Chronic Obstructive Lung Disease in Working Men in London.* New York: Oxford University Press, 1976:1–272.

Larsson C. Natural history and life expectancy in severe α1-antitrypsin deficiency, Pi Z. *Acta Med Scand* 1978;204:345–51.

O'Donnell DE, Lam M, Webb KA. Measurement of symptoms, lung hyperinflation, and endurance during exercise in chronic obstructive pulmonary disease. *Am J Respir Crit Care Med* 1998;158:1557–65.

Postma DS, Boezen HM. The natural history of chronic obstructive pulmonary disease. *Eur Respir Mon* 2006;38:71–83.

Rennard S, Thomashow B, Crapo J et al. Introducing the COPD Foundation Guide for Diagnosis and Management of COPD, recommendations of the COPD Foundation. *COPD* 2013;10:378–89.

Sandford AJ, Joos L, Paré PD. Genetic risk factors for chronic obstructive pulmonary disease. *Curr Opin Pulm Med* 2002;8:87–94.

Schols AM, Mostert R, Soeters PB, Wouters EF. Body composition and exercise performance in patients with chronic obstructive pulmonary disease. *Thorax* 1991;46:695–9.

Schols AM, Slangen J, Volovics L, Wouters EF. Weight loss is a reversible factor in the prognosis of chronic obstructive pulmonary disease. *Am J Respir Crit Care Med* 1998;157:1791–7.

Shapiro SD, Reilly Jr JJ, Rennard SI. Chronic bronchitis and emphysema. In: Mason RJ, Broadus VC, Martin TR et al., eds. *Murray & Nadel's Textbook of Respiratory Medicine*, 5th edn. Philadelphia: Elsevier, 2010:919–67.

Vestbo J, Prescott E, Lange P. Association between chronic mucus hypersecretion with FEV_1 decline and COPD morbidity. Copenhagen City Heart Study Group. *Am J Respir Crit Care Med* 1996;153:1530–5.

Symptoms

The characteristic symptom of COPD is breathlessness on exertion, sometimes accompanied by wheeze and cough, which is often, but not invariably, productive. Breathlessness is the symptom that commonly` causes the patient to seek medical attention, and it is usually the most disabling. Patients often date the onset of their illness from an episode of worsening cough with sputum production, which leaves them with a degree of chronic breathlessness. However, close questioning will often reveal the presence of a 'smoker's cough' over a period of years, along with the production of small amounts (usually < 60 mL/day) of mucoid sputum, usually predominantly in the morning.

Most patients (80%) with COPD will have a smoking history of at least 20 pack-years (1 pack-year is equivalent to smoking 20 cigarettes [1 pack] per day for 1 year or 10 a day for 2 years) before symptoms are recognized, commonly in the fifth decade. However, COPD may occur in the non-smoker and is more frequently missed in this setting.

It is characteristic of patients with COPD to progress through the clinical stages of mild, moderate and severe disease. Symptoms and signs therefore vary in any individual depending on the stage of the disease. Considerable loss of lung function can occur before symptoms become apparent, and many patients may seek medical attention when the disease is at an advanced stage, since COPD is a slowly progressive disorder and patients gradually adapt their lives to their disability. Most smokers accept cough and shortness of breath, so they often dismiss these symptoms of progressive airflow limitation as a normal consequence of their smoking habit and the aging process.

Breathlessness is the symptom that causes most disability and is associated with loss of lung function over time. In good health, the body meets the increased oxygen demand produced by exercise by using some of the inspiratory reserve volume of the lungs to increase tidal volume and by increasing respiratory rate (Figure 3.1). In COPD, because the expiratory

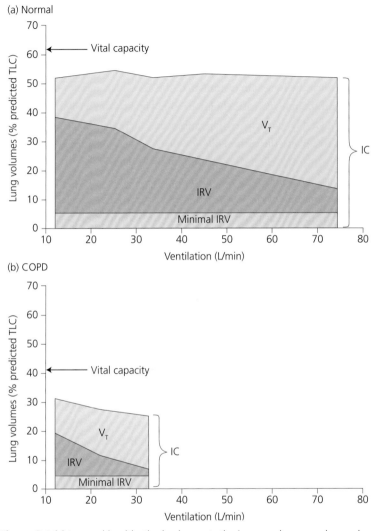

Figure 3.1 (a) In good health, the body meets the increased oxygen demand of exercise by using some of the inspiratory reserve volume (IRV) of the lungs to increase tidal volume (V_T). (b) In COPD, hyperinflation of the lungs compromises the use of IRV. The presentation of the vertical axes is inverted from normal pulmonological convention for clarity. Data from O'Donnell DE, Revill SM, Webb KA. Dynamic hyperinflation and exercise intolerance in chronic obstructive pulmonary disease. *Am J Resp Crit Care Med* 2001;164:770–7. IC, inspiratory capacity; TLC, total lung capacity.

airflow is reduced, the lungs empty slowly. As a result, the lungs become overinflated with air trapped in the alveoli, particularly when the respiratory rate increases. This hyperinflation compromises the use of the inspiratory reserve volume and breathlessness worsens. As the diaphragm flattens when the lungs are overinflated, the accessory muscles of respiration become increasingly important. The loss of alveolar/capillary surface in COPD, particularly in emphysema, increases the ventilation required to excrete the carbon dioxide that is generated during exercise, and this further increases the sensation of breathlessness.

Although breathlessness in COPD increases with exertion, it is nearly constant with time. Some patients do report variation, however; particularly that breathlessness is worse in the morning. Episodes of marked worsening, termed exacerbations, may be precipitated by acute infections. Exacerbations are distinct events and exceed the minimal day to day variation in symptoms.

Breathlessness is usually first noted while climbing hills or stairs, carrying heavy loads or hurrying on level ground. The appearance of breathlessness heralds moderate-to-severe airflow limitation. By the time the patient seeks medical advice, the forced expiratory volume in 1 second (FEV_1) has usually fallen to around 1–1.5 liters in an average man (30–45% of the expected value). Patients with COPD may adapt their breathing pattern and their behavior to minimize the sensation of breathlessness. Generally, this takes the form of greatly restricted activity.

The perception of breathlessness varies greatly between individuals with the same degree of ventilatory capacity. Breathlessness can be assessed using the modified Borg Scale (Table 3.1), a visual analog scale, the modified Medical Research Council (mMRC) Dyspnea Scale (Table 3.2), or the Dyspnea-12 scale. Mood is an important determinant of the perception of breathlessness in patients with COPD. When the FEV_1 has fallen to 30% or less of the predicted value (equivalent in an average man to an FEV_1 of around 1 liter), breathlessness is usually present on minimal exertion. Severe breathlessness is often affected by changes in temperature and by exposure to dust and fumes. Position has a variable effect on breathlessness. Some patients have severe orthopnea, relieved by leaning forward, whereas others find the greatest ease when lying flat.

TABLE 3.1

The modified Borg scale for assessing breathlessness

Scale	Severity experienced by patient
0	Nothing at all
0.5	Very, very slight (just noticeable)
1	Very slight
2	Slight (light)
3	Moderate
4	Somewhat severe
5	Severe (heavy)
6	
7	Very severe
8	
9	Very, very severe (almost maximal)
10	Maximal

TABLE 3.2

The modified Medical Research Council dyspnea scale for assessing breathlessness

Grade	Degree of breathlessness related to activities
0	Not troubled by breathlessness except on strenuous exercise
1	Short of breath when hurrying or walking up a slight hill
2	Walks slower than contemporaries on the level because of breathlessness, or has to stop for breath when walking at own pace
3	Stops for breath after walking about 100 m or after a few minutes on the level
4	Too breathless to leave the house, or breathless when dressing or undressing

Cough and sputum production. Up to 50% of cigarette smokers have a productive cough. It may either precede or appear simultaneously with the onset of breathlessness, and occurs in association with breathlessness in 75% of patients with COPD. The mMRC symptom questionnaire, which is used in epidemiological studies, employs cough as a defining symptom of chronic bronchitis, meaning a cough that produces sputum on most days for 3 consecutive months over 2 consecutive years.

Cessation of cigarette smoking produces resolution of the cough in over 90% of smokers; however, the airflow limitation often persists. Cough is often worse in the morning and, in contrast to asthma, nocturnal cough does not appear to be increased in stable COPD. In the presence of severe airway obstruction, the generation of high intrathoracic pressures may produce syncope during paroxysms of cough and 'cough fractures' of the ribs. Cough may also be exacerbated by gastroesophageal reflux.

Sputum production is a common, though not universal, feature of COPD. Sputum is usually white or gray in color, but may become mucopurulent and green or yellow in color during exacerbations. However, some patients with COPD have persistently purulent sputum; this may relate to bacterial colonization in the airway. Indeed, it is now recognized that a number of such patients have underlying bronchiectasis. Excessive sputum production (more than 60 mL/day) should raise the possibility of bronchiectasis.

Hemoptysis can occur in exacerbations of COPD in association with infection, but should always be treated seriously, since the incidence of bronchial carcinoma is high in patients with COPD. The production of copious amounts of frothy sputum, particularly in association with orthopnea or hypertension and/or ischemic heart disease, raises the possibility of left ventricular failure and pulmonary edema.

Wheeze is common in COPD, but is not universally present and is a non-specific symptom. It is not easy to evaluate because of its intermittent nature and the difficulties patients experience in understanding this symptom. Wheeze is due to turbulent airflow through the larger airways as a result of various causes including bronchial smooth muscle contraction, structural airway narrowing and the presence of excess airway secretions. Wheeze does not usually wake patients with COPD at night as it does those with asthma. The absence of signs of wheeze on auscultation of the chest does not exclude a diagnosis of COPD.

Other symptoms. Chest pain is common in patients with COPD, but is often unrelated to the disease itself, and may be due to underlying ischemic heart disease or gastroesophageal reflux. Patients with COPD often complain of chest tightness during exacerbations of breathlessness, particularly during exercise, and this is sometimes difficult to distinguish from ischemic cardiac pain. Pleuritic chest pain may suggest an intercurrent pneumothorax, pneumonia or pulmonary infarction.

Weight loss is a feature of severe COPD and is thought to result from anorexia, decreased calorie intake and increased metabolism.

Psychiatric morbidity, particularly depression, is common in patients with severe COPD, which is likely to reflect the social isolation and the chronicity of the disease. Sleep quality is impaired in advanced COPD, which may contribute to the impaired neuropsychiatric performance.

History

A detailed history is important in COPD and should include:

- full smoking history
- exposure to other risk factors, particularly gases or dusts, and an occupational history
- medical history including asthma, allergy, sinusitis, nasal polyps, respiratory infection in childhood and other respiratory diseases
- family history of COPD or other chronic respiratory disease
- symptom development
- exacerbations or previous hospitalizations for respiratory disorders
- presence of comorbidity
- appropriateness of current medical treatment
- effect of the disease on the patient's life, including limitation of activity, work days lost and economic impact, effect on family and feelings of depression or anxiety
- social and family support available to the patient.

As well as comorbidities commonly associated with COPD that should be addressed in their own right, the patient may have comorbidities such as heart disease that may further contribute to the restriction of activity (Table 3.3).

COPD is most common among smokers and after the age of 40. The presence of symptoms or signs in non-smokers or in younger individuals does not exclude COPD, but should raise suspicion of another condition and lead to a review of the other possible diagnoses or increased genetic susceptibility to COPD, such as α1-antitrypsin deficiency (see page 28). Importantly, there is, in general, a dose–response relationship between the number of cigarettes smoked and the FEV_1; however, huge individual variations (see Figure 2.1) reflect the varying susceptibility to cigarette smoke.

Occupational exposure to dusts has an additive effect on the decline in lung function. This has particularly been shown in coal miners in whom both smoking and years of dust exposure contribute to the decline in FEV_1. Similar additive effects have been observed with air pollution. The contribution of smoking, however, is three times as great as that of dust exposure in miners.

TABLE 3.3

Systemic effects and comorbidities in COPD

• Cardiac	• Skeletal muscle weakness
– Infarction	• Skin wrinkling
– Arrhythmia	• Diabetes mellitus
– Heart failure	• Glaucoma
• Hypercoagulability	• Peptic ulceration
– Stroke	• Gastroesophageal reflux
– Deep vein thrombosis	• Anemia
– Pulmonary embolism	• Fluid retention
• Aortic aneurysm	• Depression
• Osteoporosis	• Lung cancer
• Weight loss	

Physical signs

The physical signs seen in patients with COPD are not specific to the disease. They depend on the degree of airflow limitation and pulmonary overinflation, and may be virtually absent in patients with mild-to-moderate disease, so their sensitivity in detecting or excluding COPD is poor. Physical signs of airflow limitation are rarely present until lung function is significantly impaired. Detection of early COPD is possible only by spirometry or by imaging techniques, such as high-resolution computed tomography (HRCT) to detect emphysema.

Breathing pattern. Patients with COPD often have a characteristic breathing pattern with a prolonged expiratory phase, although this is usually present only when disease is severe. Some patients adopt pursed-lipped breathing on expiration, which may reduce expiratory airway collapse. The use of the accessory muscles of respiration, particularly the sternomastoids, is often seen in advanced disease; these patients often lean forward, supporting themselves with their arms to fix the shoulder girdle, thus allowing the use of the pectorals and the latissimus dorsi to increase chest wall movement.

Signs of overinflation include:

- increased anterior/posterior diameter of the chest, which when greater than the lateral diameter is described as a 'barrel-shaped chest'
- horizontal ribs with prominent sternal angle and wide subcostal angle
- reduced distance between the suprasternal notch and the cricoid cartilage (normally three finger-breadths)
- inspiratory tracheal tug
- Hoover's sign, which is when the horizontal position of the diaphragm acts to pull in the lower ribs during inspiration
- increased intrathoracic pressure swings, which may result in indrawing of the suprasternal and supraclavicular fossae and the intercostal muscles
- decreased hepatic and cardiac dullness on percussion of the chest; the absence of a dull percussion note, normally due to the underlying heart, over the lower end of the sternum, is a useful sign of gross overinflation.

Breath sounds may have a prolonged expiratory phase, or may be uniformly diminished, particularly in the advanced stages of the disease. Wheeze may be heard by the unaided ear, at the patient's mouth if necessary, and may be variably present on auscultation both on inspiration and expiration. Crackles may be present, particularly at the lung bases, but are usually scanty, vary with coughing and cannot be distinguished from the coarse crackles of bronchiectasis or the fine respiratory crackles of fibrosis or left ventricular failure.

Different degrees of tachypnea may be present in patients with severe COPD, and prolonged forced expiratory time (> 5 seconds) can be a useful indicator of airway obstruction.

Physical appearance. In advanced disease, cyanosis may be present, indicating hypoxemia, but may be influenced by the background lighting or accentuated by polycythemia, and therefore is a fairly subjective sign. The flapping tremor associated with hypercapnia is neither sensitive nor specific, and the often reported papilledema associated with severe hypercapnia is in fact rarely seen.

Weight loss may be apparent in advanced disease, as well as a reduction in muscle mass.

Finger clubbing is not a manifestation of COPD and should suggest the possibility of complicating bronchial neoplasm, bronchiectasis or lung fibrosis.

Cardiovascular signs. Overinflation of the chest makes it difficult to locate the apex beat and reduces the cardiac dullness. The characteristic signs indicative of the presence or consequences of pulmonary arterial hypertension may be difficult to detect in advanced disease. The heave of right ventricular hypertrophy may be palpable at the lower left sternal edge or in the subcostal angle. Heart sounds are generally soft, though the second heart sound may be exaggerated in the second left intercostal space in the presence of pulmonary hypertension. Splitting of the second heart sound with an increased pulmonary component may be present. There may be a right-sided gallop rhythm, with a third sound audible in the fourth intercostal space to the left of the sternum or in the epigastrium.

The jugular venous pressure can be difficult to assess in patients with COPD as it varies widely with respiration and is difficult to discern because of the prominent accessory muscle activity. When the fluid retention of cor pulmonale occurs, there may be evidence of functional tricuspid incompetence, producing a pansystolic murmur at the left sternal edge.

Peripheral vasodilation accompanies hypercapnia, producing warm peripheries with a high-volume pulse. Pitting peripheral edema may be present as a result of fluid retention. However, other causes of edema, such as venous stasis, low serum albumin and deep venous thrombosis, should be considered.

Hepatic signs. The liver may be tender and pulsatile, and a prominent 'v' wave may be visible in the jugular venous pulse. The liver may also be palpable below the right costal margin as a result of the low diaphragm due to overinflation of the lungs.

Skin signs. Wrinkling of the skin has been associated with the presence of emphysema.

Clinical presentation

Many smokers accept the development of exertional dyspnea and cough with sputum production as an inevitable consequence of the smoking habit, and therefore often present to their doctor when the disease is at a fairly advanced stage. Relatively few patients are diagnosed early in the course of the disease. All smokers should quit. However, repeated spirometry over the course of several years will identify smokers with a rapid decline in FEV_1 whose function may still be normal, who could be targeted for smoking cessation and early therapeutic intervention.

Some patients present initially to hospital or to their primary care provider during an exacerbation of the disease and claim that they had no significant symptoms until that time. However, close questioning often reveals the presence of progressive symptoms.

Two clinical patterns have been described, both of which represent severe disease – the so-called 'pink puffers' and 'blue bloaters'. The pink and puffing patient is thin and breathless with blood gas values that are preserved until late in the course of the disease, and therefore does not

43

develop pulmonary hypertension until the disease is very advanced. By contrast, the blue and bloated patient develops hypoxemia and hypercapnia earlier, and thus also the complications of edema and secondary polycythemia. These 'phenotypes' are not indicative of emphysema or bronchitis, as was once thought, but clearly indicate the varied systemic manifestations of COPD. These subtypes of COPD, however, only partially capture the heterogeneity of the diseases. Most patients lie between these two extremes, and many patients fit neither pattern.

Systemic effects and comorbidities

Traditionally, COPD is regarded as a disease of the lungs characterized by progressive symptoms and a decline in lung function. Therapeutic strategies such as bronchodilators and inhaled glucocorticosteroids have therefore been used for relieving symptoms in association with improving airflow limitation. However, COPD is also associated with a number of systemic effects and common comorbidities (see Table 3.3), which may be present at any stage of the disease. Some of these comorbidities arise independent of COPD, whereas others appear to be causally related, either as a result of shared risk factors or the influence of COPD on the development of another condition. Systemic inflammation in COPD may be the link between COPD and some of its comorbidities.

Comorbid conditions have an important effect on morbidity and mortality, and should be comprehensively assessed and managed in all patients with COPD. In general, comorbidities should be treated in the same way as in patients without COPD.

Skeletal muscle dysfunction. Exercise limitation is a common complaint in COPD and is usually explained on the basis of the increased work of breathing caused by airflow limitation. However, almost 50% of patients with COPD stop exercising because of leg fatigue, not because of breathlessness. This suggests that skeletal muscle dysfunction is an important factor in the symptom complex. Skeletal muscle dysfunction is a good predictor of poor exercise performance, correlating more strongly than either lung function or blood gas measurements. This dysfunction is not entirely caused by a sedentary lifestyle, but the mechanisms involved are not yet fully understood; limited oxygen delivery or cellular changes in the skeletal muscle due to the inflammatory processes underlying COPD may be implicated.

Weight loss is experienced by many patients with COPD during the course of their disease (see Figure 2.4). This phenomenon is of prognostic value, and is independent of the more traditional prognostic factors related to FEV_1 and the partial pressure of oxygen in arterial blood (PaO_2).

The mechanisms underlying the weight loss are unclear, but may be related to the increased metabolic rate, tissue hypoxia and systemic inflammation.

Cardiovascular disease is the most common and probably the most important comorbidity in patients with COPD. General population studies and studies in patients with COPD suggest that COPD is an important risk factor for ischemic heart disease and sudden cardiac death. Indeed, the FEV_1 is an established predictor of cardiovascular mortality. Ischemic heart disease and myocardial infarction are underdiagnosed and consequently are often undertreated in patients with COPD. The mechanism responsible for the increased risk of cardiovascular disease in patients with COPD is unknown, but hypotheses include the effect of systemic inflammation and vascular dysfunction.

Heart failure occurs in around 30% of patients with stable COPD and is an important differential diagnosis in exacerbations of COPD. Compromise of ventricular filling, in part due to hyperinflation, and compromise of the pulmonary circulation may contribute to diastolic dysfunction.

Hypertension is the most frequent comorbidity in COPD and has an adverse effect on prognosis.

Osteoporosis is more common in patients with COPD than in the general population. This may be due, in part, to concurrent smoking and to the use of corticosteroids. COPD itself appears to be associated with bone mineral loss and there is a particular association with emphysema and a low body mass index.

Psychiatric problems, particularly depression and anxiety, are common among patients with COPD and are associated with a poor prognosis. Studies suggest that both prevalent and incident depression is more common among patients with COPD than among similarly aged individuals with other diseases of similar morbidity. Anxiety and depression in patients with COPD are associated with younger age, female sex, greater airflow limitation, reduced health-related quality of life and a history of cardiovascular disease.

Diabetes and the metabolic syndrome are more common in patients with COPD than the general population and the presence of diabetes has an adverse effect on prognosis.

Lung cancer. COPD, in particular emphysema, also increases the risk of lung cancer, which is the commonest cause of death in patients with mild airflow limitation. The mechanism is again unclear, but may result from common risk factors such as smoking, the involvement of susceptibility genes or failure to clear carcinogens.

Other respiratory conditions. With the increased use of CT scanning, bronchiectasis is increasingly recognized in patients with COPD and is associated with longer exacerbations and a poor prognosis.

A significant proportion of patients with chronic airflow limitation have features suggestive of both COPD and asthma. The term 'asthma COPD overlap syndrome (ACOS)' has been used to describe these patients. The prevalence of this syndrome is estimated to be between 15% and 50% of patients depending on the defining criteria. There are no recognized defining features for ACOS, but patients with features of both COPD and asthma have poor health-related quality of life, frequent exacerbations, a more rapid decline in lung function and a higher mortality.

Systemic inflammation. COPD is characterized by an excessive inflammatory process in the lung parenchyma in response to inhaled particles or gases. Evidence of inflammation has also been detected in the systemic circulation, such as markers of oxidative stress, elevated levels of cytokines and activation of circulating leukocytes. Systemic inflammation has been associated with some COPD comorbidities and a poor prognosis.

Spectrum of disease

Many national and international guidelines for COPD have used a simple classification of disease severity based on spirometry. However, because FEV_1 only partially captures the severity of COPD, recent recommendations suggest assessing additional measures. The most recent classification from the Global initiative for chronic Obstructive Lung Disease (GOLD) takes into account symptoms and exacerbation risk in addition to airflow limitation (Figure 3.2). First, the patient's symptoms are assessed using the COPD assessment test (CAT) or the modified MRC score (mMRC) for dyspnea (see Table 3.2). The CAT is the preferred test as it provides a comprehensive assessment of symptoms

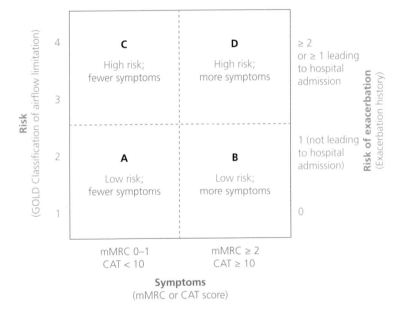

Figure 3.2 Patients can be classified into groups A, B, C or D after assessment of COPD that takes into account symptoms, degree of airflow limitation using spirometry and risk of exacerbations. The highest risk according to the GOLD grade or exacerbation history should be used (≥ 1 hospitalization for a COPD exacerbation should be considered high risk). CAT, COPD assessment test; mMRC, modified Medical Research Council dyspnea scale (see Table 3.2). Reproduced with permission from the *Global Strategy for the Diagnosis, Management and Prevention of COPD*, GOLD 2016. www.goldcopd.org.

(www.catestonline.org). A CAT score of 10 or more indicates a high level of symptoms. Exacerbation risk is then assessed in three ways: by the severity of airflow limitation as indicated by spirometry grade, with a GOLD classification of 3 or 4 indicating high risk (see Table 4.1); by the patient's history of exacerbations, with two or more exacerbations in the preceding year indicating high risk; and by the patient's history of hospitalization in the preceding year. The highest risk parameter should be recorded for the purposes of this assessment. Alternatively, the COPD Foundation Guide recommends assessing seven independent domains of severity (Table 3.4).

Key points – clinical features

- COPD occurs, though less commonly, in those who do not smoke.
- Usually (in 80% of patients) there is a significant smoking history of at least 20 pack-years. For those with lesser smoking histories or for younger individuals, consider an alternative diagnosis or a genetic predisposition (e.g. α1-antitrypsin deficiency).
- The most common symptom in COPD is breathlessness on exertion.
- Dyspnea may be discounted by patients until disease is severe, as breathlessness can be avoided by restricting activity.
- Physical signs often present only at an advanced stage of the disease.
- Clinical indicators include signs of overinflation, prominent use of accessory muscles of respiration, weight loss, expiratory wheeze, cyanosis, peripheral edema and raised jugular venous pressure. These are usually apparent only in severe disease.
- The systemic effects of COPD result in a number of comorbidities that impact on the morbidity and mortality of the disease.
- The full spectrum of COPD can now be better identified using new classifications of disease that take into account symptoms and exacerbation risk in addition to airflow limitation.

TABLE 3.4

Domains for clinical assessment in COPD

- Airflow (FEV_1)

- Symptoms (CAT or mMRC dyspnea scale)

- Exacerbation history

- Oxygenation

- Emphysema

- Chronic bronchitis

- Comorbidities

CAT, COPD assessment test (www.catestonline.org); FEV_1, forced expiratory volume in 1 second; mMRC, modified Medical Research Council (see Table 3.2). Source: COPD Foundation. www.copdfoundation.org, last accessed 19 January 2016.

Key references

Agusti AGN. Systemic effects of COPD. *Proc Am Thorac Soc* 2007;4:522–5.

American Thoracic Society and European Respiratory Society. Skeletal muscle dysfunction in chronic obstructive pulmonary disease. *Am J Respir Crit Care Med* 1999;159:S1–40.

Calverley PM, Georgopoulos D. Chronic obstructive pulmonary disease: symptoms and signs. *Eur Respir Mon* 2006;38:7–23.

Fabbri LM, Luppi F, Beghé B, Rabe KF. Complex comorbidities of COPD. *Eur Respir J* 2008;31: 204–12.

MacNee W. Chronic bronchitis and emphysema. In: Seaton A, Seaton D, Leitch AG, eds. *Crofton and Douglas's Respiratory Diseases*, 5th edn. Oxford: Blackwell Science, 2000:616–95.

Rennard S, Thomashow B, Crapo J et al. Introducing the COPD Foundation Guide for Diagnosis and Management of COPD, recommendations of the COPD Foundation. *COPD* 2013:10; 378–89.

Soriano JB, Visick GT, Muellerova H et al. Patterns of comorbidities in newly diagnosed COPD and asthma in primary care. *Chest* 2005;128:2099–107.

Spirometry

The most important disturbance of respiratory function in COPD is obstruction to forced expiratory flow. The degree of airflow obstruction cannot be predicted from the symptoms and signs, and therefore assessment of the degree and the progression of airway obstruction should be encouraged in both primary and secondary care. To identify patients early in the course of the disease, spirometry should be performed for those who have chronic cough and sputum production, and for those at risk, such as smokers, even if they have no dyspnea. In the early stages of the disease, conventional spirometry may reveal no abnormality. This is because the earliest changes in COPD affect the alveolar walls and small airways. The resulting modest increase in peripheral airway resistance is not reflected in the conventional spirometric measurements. A reduction in forced expiratory volume in 1 second (FEV_1) relative to vital capacity may, however, be a more sensitive measure. Similarly, sequential measures, which track changes in lung function, may also be more sensitive indicators. Serial measures in at-risk individuals can demonstrate loss of function even if the measurements themselves are still in the normal range.

Diagnosing COPD using spirometry. Spirometry is the most robust test of airflow limitation in patients with COPD. Spirometry assesses the volume of exhaled air over time and is performed with the patient exhaling from a maximum inhalation to a maximum exhalation using maximum force to blow out all the air as hard and as fast as possible. In healthy individuals, this forced expiratory maneuver can be completed in 3–4 seconds but, in patients with increasing airflow limitation, it may take up to 15 seconds. The volume of air exhaled is plotted on a graph against the time taken to reach the maximum exhalation (Figure 4.1). Three indices can then be derived:

- forced expiratory volume in 1 second (FEV_1)
- forced vital capacity (FVC), which is the total volume of air that can be exhaled from a maximum inhalation to a maximum exhalation
- the ratio of FEV_1 to FVC, expressed as a percentage.

Figure 4.1 Normal spirometry. FEV$_1$, forced expiratory volume in 1 second; FVC, forced vital capacity.

FEV$_1$ and FVC are expressed in absolute values in liters and also as a percentage of the predicted values for the individual depending on their age, height, sex and ethnic origin. Values within ± 20% of the predicted values are considered to be within the normal range. Thus, an FEV$_1$ of over 80% of the predicted value is considered to be normal. Under normal circumstances, 70–80% of the total volume of the air in the lungs (the FVC) should be exhaled in the first second. In other words, the FEV$_1$:FVC ratio is normally 0.7–0.8. When airflow through the airways is obstructed, it is not possible to exhale so much air in the first second, and the FEV$_1$:FVC ratio falls. A ratio of less than 0.7 indicates airflow obstruction (Figure 4.2). A post-bronchodilator FEV$_1$:FVC ratio below 0.7 indicates chronic airflow limitation and is a diagnostic criterion for COPD.

The use of a fixed FEV$_1$:FVC ratio as a diagnostic criterion for chronic airflow limitation is a pragmatic approach, as reference values for FEV$_1$:FVC are unavailable. However, the fixed ratio has limitations because the ratio declines with age, with the potential for overdiagnosis of COPD in the elderly. It also has the potential to underdiagnose disease in younger individuals. The lower limit of normal (LLN) is an alternative approach to the fixed ratio to determine the presence of COPD. The LLN threshold is defined as the fifth percentile of the normal population

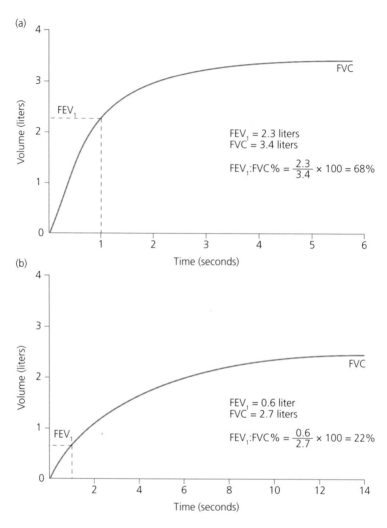

Figure 4.2 (a) Spirometry showing mild obstruction. (b) Spirometry showing severe obstruction. Note the different time range of the x-axes. FEV_1, forced expiratory volume in 1 second; FVC, forced vital capacity.

distribution of FEV_1/FVC. If an individual's FEV_1:FVC falls below this fifth percentile, the individual is defined as having COPD.

It should be noted that the pathological conditions of emphysema and chronic bronchitis can be present despite a normal FEV_1:FVC ratio. Thus, normal spirometric values do not exclude the presence of disease.

In airway obstruction, the FEV_1 is reduced both in terms of volume and as a percentage of the predicted value. The FVC also falls, but less than the FEV_1, so that the FEV_1:FVC ratio decreases (see Figure 4.2). By contrast, in restrictive defects, such as lung fibrosis or chest-wall deformity, the airway size remains normal, but both the FEV_1 and FVC are reduced, so the ratio remains above 0.7 (Figure 4.3).

Classification of severity. Patients with COPD typically show a decrease in both the FEV_1 and the FEV_1:FVC ratio (the latter being a more sensitive measure of early airflow limitation). The degree of spirometric abnormality generally reflects the severity of COPD and is used as part of the classification. The spirometric severity classification defined by the Global initiative for chronic Obstructive Lung Disease (GOLD) is based on post-bronchodilator spirometry (Table 4.1), and is most widely used for research purposes. The COPD Foundation proposes a slightly simpler severity classification for clinical implementation, based on the recommendations of the American Clinical Society, which provides a more complete classification of spirometric results (Figure 4.4).

Figure 4.3 Spirometry showing a restrictive defect; the FEV_1:FVC ratio is within the normal range. FEV_1, forced expiratory volume in 1 second; FVC, forced vital capacity.

TABLE 4.1

GOLD classification of the severity of airflow limitation

Stage	Characteristics
I: Mild	FEV_1:FVC < 70%
	FEV_1 ≥ 80% predicted
II: Moderate	FEV_1:FVC < 70%
	50% ≤ FEV_1 < 80% predicted
III: Severe	FEV_1:FVC < 70%
	30% ≤ FEV_1 < 50% predicted
IV: Very severe	FEV_1:FVC < 70%
	FEV_1 < 30% predicted

FEV_1, post-bronchodilator forced expiratory volume in 1 second; FVC, forced vital capacity; GOLD, Global initiative for chronic Obstructive Lung Disease.

Reproduced with permission from the *Global Strategy for the Diagnosis, Management, and Prevention of Chronic Obstructive Pulmonary Disease*. Global Initiative for Chronic Obstructive Lung Disease (GOLD) 2016. www.goldcopd.org

Spirometry alone does not provide a complete assessment of severity, particularly with respect to functional status. In addition to spirometry, assessment of severity should include symptoms, presence of exacerbations, oxygenation, emphysema, chronic bronchitis, and presence of comorbidities (see Table 3.4). Several approaches have been adopted that combine various features into a single measure of COPD severity. For example, the BODE index (Body mass index, Obstruction, Dyspnea, Exercise; Table 4.2) is a better predictor of mortality than any individual variable alone, while the CAT (COPD assessment test) is a unidimensional measure of health status with a focus on symptoms, which has been validated as an index of clinical worsening over time (see pages 47–8).

Technique. It is important that a volume plateau is reached in spirometry. This can take 15 seconds or more in a patient with severe airway obstruction. If this maneuver is not carried out properly, the FVC can be underestimated. Many spirometers currently in use substitute the forced expiratory volume in 6 seconds for FVC. Such instruments therefore

- **SG-0 Normal spirometry**; does not rule out emphysema, chronic bronchitis, asthma or risk of developing exacerbations or COPD
- **SG-1 Mild COPD** Post-bronchodilator FEV_1/FVC ratio < 0.7, FEV_1 > 60% predicted
- **SG-2 Moderate COPD** Post-bronchodilator FEV_1/FVC ratio < 0.7, > 30% predicted
- **SG-3 Severe COPD** Post-bronchodilator FEV_1/FVC ratio < 0.7, FEV_1 < 30% predicted
- **SG-U Undefined** FEV_1/FVC ratio > 0.7, FEV_1 < 80% predicted; consistent with restriction, muscle weakness and other pathologies

Figure 4.4 Classification of spirometric findings (COPD Foundation Guide). Start by determining the patient's symptoms, as represented by the COPD assessment test (CAT; www.catestonline.org) and/or modified Medical Research Council (mMRC) questionnaire (see Table 3.2). Next, look at the patient's risk by comparing spirometry readings and exacerbation history. The highest risk parameter should always be recorded to yield a more accurate reflection of the patient's current COPD status.

underestimate the vital capacity, and thus yield artificially elevated $FEV_1:FVC$ ratios. This limitation is not felt to be a major impediment for the diagnosis of COPD (the criterion being a ratio < 0.7), but it does reduce the reliability of the ratio as a gauge of disease severity.

Since FEV_1 is effort-dependent, traces should be checked to ensure that maximum effort has been achieved and that full expiration has been performed. The FEV_1 is very reproducible and varies by less than 170 mL between maneuvers if the test is carried out correctly. The test reproducibility is an excellent measure of the effort exerted by the patient and the quality of the test. In contrast to maximal efforts, which are highly reproducible, submaximal efforts are highly variable. Therefore, reproducibility of the tests to within ± 2% is generally regarded as a

TABLE 4.2

Variables and point values used for the computation of the BODE index

Variable	Points on BODE index			
	0	1	2	3
FEV$_1$ (% of predicted)	≥ 65	50–64	36–49	≤ 35
Distance walked in 6 minutes (m)	≥ 350	250–349	150–249	≤ 149
mMRC dyspnea scale*	0–1	2	3	4
Body mass index	> 21	≤ 21		

*See Table 3.2. BODE, body mass index, degree of airflow obstruction and dyspnea, and exercise capacity; FEV$_1$, forced expiratory volume in 1 second; mMRC, modified Medical Research Council.

measure of satisfactory test quality; many modern spirometers can perform such assessments automatically.

The FVC also depends on effort, particularly during the latter part of the maneuver, and results are more variable. To avoid the effect of airway collapse in patients with COPD during a forced expiratory maneuver, it is suggested that a relaxed or slow vital capacity (VC) measurement, in which the patient exhales at his/her own pace after maximum inhalation, should be used. The slow VC is often 0.5 liters greater than the FVC. With increasing airflow obstruction, it takes longer to exhale and the early slope of the volume–time trace becomes less steep (see Figure 4.2b).

In assessing FEV$_1$, the following points should be remembered.
- Patients should be clinically stable (i.e. at least 4 weeks must have passed since the last exacerbation) to establish 'baseline' lung function.
- If patients have taken a bronchodilator, results may be improved from 'baseline'.
- Patients should be sitting in an upright position.
- An adequate explanation of the technique should be given.
- Patients should be asked to take a maximum breath in and then place their lips around the mouthpiece, forming an airtight seal.

- Patients should then be encouraged to exhale as hard, as fast and as completely as possible.
- Adequate time should be allowed for recovery between exhalations, with a maximum of six forced maneuvers being performed in one session.
- Three technically satisfactory maneuvers giving similar results should be carried out.
- At least two readings of FEV_1 should be within 100 mL or 5% of each other.

Peak expiratory flow

Peak expiratory flow (PEF) can either be read directly from the flow–volume loop (see page 60) or measured with a handheld peak flow meter. It is a simple, quick and inexpensive way of measuring airflow obstruction, and has been particularly useful for repeated measurements in patients with asthma to reveal spontaneous diurnal variation or variations in response to therapy. The PEF meter measures the maximal flow rate that can be maintained over 10 ms; it is most effective for monitoring changes in airflow in an individual over time, but should not be used in the diagnosis of COPD. In COPD, there is little daily change in PEF and many of the variations are often within the error range of the measurement. Although repeated measurements of PEF can replace measurement of FEV_1, single measurements are not as useful as the variation is so high. There are several theoretical reasons why FEV_1 is a better measurement than PEF in the diagnosis and assessment of COPD (Table 4.3). However, for clinicians who lack office spirometry, performance of a PEF may be useful in deciding whom to refer for the more definitive testing needed for diagnosis.

Bronchodilator reversibility testing

The main objectives of a bronchodilator reversibility test in COPD are:

- to help distinguish those patients with marked reversibility who have underlying asthma (it is the post-bronchodilator lung function that defines the presence and severity of airflow limitation in COPD)
- to establish the post-bronchodilator FEV_1, which is the best predictor of long-term prognosis
- to establish the best obtainable lung function.

TABLE 4.3

Reasons why FEV$_1$ is the measurement of choice in COPD

- It is a reproducible and objective measurement. There are well-defined normal ranges that allow for the effects of age, race and sex
- It is relatively simple and quick to measure and can be measured at all stages of disease
- The forced expiratory maneuver records not only FEV$_1$, but also FVC. An FEV$_1$:FVC ratio < 70% is diagnostic of airway obstruction. If the ratio is normal (> 70%) and the test was performed well, the pattern is not obstructive and the diagnosis is not COPD
- PEF measurements cannot determine whether values are low because of obstruction or restriction
- The variance of repeated FEV$_1$ measurements in the same person is well documented and is low
- Studies of mortality and disability have shown that the FEV$_1$ predicts future mortality from COPD and other respiratory and cardiac diseases
- Serial measurements provide evidence of disease progression
- In COPD, the relationship between PEF and FEV$_1$ is poor
- PEF may underestimate the degree of airway obstruction in COPD
- FEV$_1$ is better related to prognosis and disability than FEV$_1$:FVC ratio, because the FVC depends on effort and is therefore more variable

FEV$_1$, forced expiratory volume in 1 second; FVC, forced vital capacity; PEF, peak expiratory flow.

There is no agreement on a standardized method of assessing reversibility. Usually changes in the FEV$_1$ or PEF are monitored, but reversibility could also be determined as a change in static lung volumes after administration of a bronchodilator.

The use of bronchodilator testing in patients with COPD is limited by the variability of the FEV$_1$ measurement itself, and by the fact that, by definition, patients with COPD may have only a small degree of reversibility, which is often within the error of the measurement. Bronchodilator reversibility tests can also vary from day to day depending on the degree of bronchomotor tone. A change in FEV$_1$ that exceeds 170 mL can be considered not to have occurred by chance. Most guidelines recommend that changes should be considered significant only if they exceed 200 mL. In addition to this absolute change in FEV_1, a percentage change of 12% over baseline has been suggested as significant in the American Thoracic Society and the GOLD guidelines, whereas an improvement of 15% over baseline FEV_1 and a 200 mL absolute change is recommended in the European Respiratory Society and British Thoracic Society guidelines.

Reversibility testing with a bronchodilator is generally indicated only at the time of diagnosis. Bronchodilator testing should usually be undertaken only in patients with COPD at stage II (moderate) and above, and reversibility testing should be conducted during a period of clinical stability, with a high dose of bronchodilator in order not to miss a significant response. The high dose can be delivered by means of a nebulizer. An alternative method is to deliver a smaller dose of the drug by giving repeated doses from a metered-dose inhaler through a large-volume spacer. The usual recommended protocol for testing bronchial reversibility is shown in Table 4.4. Improvement of lung function to normal suggests a diagnosis of asthma without the presence of COPD.

Daily variations in airway smooth muscle tone may affect the response to bronchodilators in patients with COPD. Thus, when airway smooth muscle tone is higher and FEV_1 is therefore lower, a response to bronchodilators may be more likely than when muscle tone is lower and

---

TABLE 4.4

Guidelines for bronchodilator reversibility testing

- Withhold all bronchodilators for sufficient time for therapeutic effect to abate
- Record FEV_1 before and 15 minutes after giving salbutamol (albuterol)*, 2.5–5 mg, or nebulized terbutaline, 5–10 mg
- Record (preferably on a separate occasion) FEV_1 before and 30 minutes after nebulized ipratropium bromide, 500 µg
- Record (on a separate occasion) FEV_1 before and 30 minutes after a combination of salbutamol (albuterol) or terbutaline and ipratropium

*Salbutamol is the recommended international non-proprietary name favored by the World Health Organization; albuterol is the official generic name in the USA.
FEV_1, forced expiratory volume in 1 second.

FEV$_1$ higher. One-third of those patients who are initially shown to have a response to a bronchodilator may, on retesting on a different day, have no response. Conversely, patients who do not show a significant FEV$_1$ response to a bronchodilator can still benefit symptomatically from long-term bronchodilator treatment. Therefore, 'significant' reversibility does not predict clinical response to bronchodilators, perhaps because dynamic hyperinflation drives symptoms. Treatment of patients with COPD with bronchodilators is guided by clinical response, not by spirometry.

In patients with COPD, bronchodilator reversibility testing or small changes in FEV$_1$ over time are predictive of disease progression or response to treatment. However, larger changes (> 400 mL) are suggestive of asthma.

Specialized lung function tests

Flow–volume loops. Many spirometers plot expiratory flow rate throughout the entire expiration at the same time as a standard volume–time trace. The PEF, which is sustained for 10 ms, represents the flow only in the larger airways. However, the flow–volume trace interprets flow from all generations of the airways and may be more helpful than PEF in detecting early airway narrowing in smaller airways (Figure 4.5).

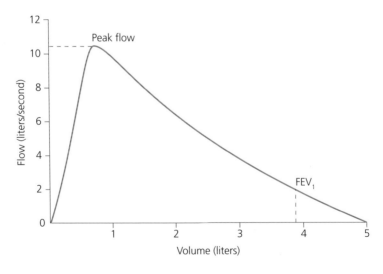

Figure 4.5 Normal flow–volume curve.

Expiratory flow rates at 75% or 50% of VC have been used as a measure of airflow limitation, and provide complementary information to that obtained from the usual volume–time plot. There are problems with the reproducibility of these measurements, so that values must fall below 50% of the predicted values to be considered abnormal. Flows at lung volumes below 50% of VC were previously considered to be an indicator of small-airways dysfunction, but probably provide no more clinically useful information than measurement of FEV_1. Examples of flow–volume loops in airflow obstruction are shown in Figure 4.6.

The flow–volume loop can also help to identify the presence of obstruction of the large airways. The patterns of obstruction can vary with inspiration and expiration.

Lung volumes. Measurements of static lung volumes, such as total lung capacity, residual volume and functional residual capacity (Figure 4.7), can be made using a body plethysmograph or the helium dilution technique. These measurements are used to assess the degree of overinflation and gas trapping resulting from loss of elastic recoil and collapse of the airways. It is known that dynamic overinflation occurs in COPD, particularly during exercise, and it may be an important determinant of symptoms such as breathlessness. Inspiratory capacity may be a useful surrogate for more precise measures of dynamic hyperinflation (see Figure 3.1).

The standard method for measuring static lung volumes using the helium dilution technique during rebreathing may underestimate lung volumes, particularly in patients with bullous disease, where the inspired helium does not have time to equilibrate properly in the airspaces. The body plethysmograph uses Boyle's law to calculate lung volumes from measurements of changes in mouth and body plethysmograph pressures during gentle panting against a closed shutter. This technique measures trapped air within the thorax and thus includes poorly ventilated areas, which therefore gives higher measurements than the helium dilution technique in COPD. CT scans on inhalation/exhalation can also be used to measure lung volumes.

Gas transfer by the lungs can be measured using carbon monoxide as a tracer gas. Following inhalation of a small amount of carbon monoxide,

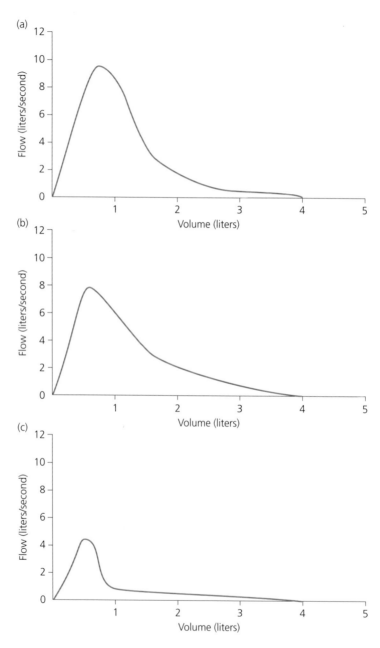

Figure 4.6 Examples of flow–volume curves. (a) Mild obstruction. (b) Moderate obstruction. (c) Severe obstruction.

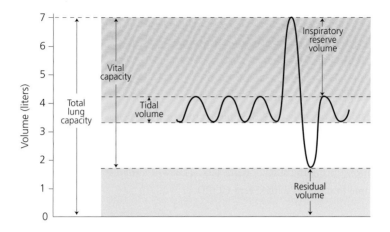

Figure 4.7 Lung volume measurements.

some of the inhaled marker is transferred from the lungs into the pulmonary capillary blood where it binds to hemoglobin. Reductions in the concentration of carbon monoxide in the exhaled gas can therefore be used to gauge the efficiency of gas transfer within the lung. Some of the reduction in carbon monoxide level is also due to diffusion into the residual volume of the lung. Thus, values for the diffusing capacity in the lung for carbon monoxide (DLco; TLco in the UK) are generally corrected using helium, which diffuses into the residual volume but is not absorbed into the pulmonary capillary blood. This technique yields the ventilated alveolar volume (V_A), which provides the carbon monoxide transfer coefficient Kco (DLco/V_A).

DLco values are normal in asthma, but below normal in many patients with COPD. Although there is a relationship between the DLco and the extent of emphysema, the severity of the emphysema in an individual patient cannot be predicted from the DLco. Neither is a low DLco specific for emphysema, as it can be affected by cigarette smoking, anemia and lung diseases, such as pulmonary fibrosis and pulmonary thromboembolism. Thus a low DLco in a patient with COPD suggests a significant degree of alveolar destruction, probably as a result of emphysema, but a normal DLco does not exclude a diagnosis of COPD. The DLco is sometimes helpful in patients with breathlessness that is out of proportion to the degree of airflow limitation.

The principal factors affecting the DLco are:

- the thickness of the alveolar membrane
- capillary blood volume
- hemoglobin concentration (the test needs to be corrected for hemoglobin concentration).

The most widely used method for measuring DLco is the single-breath technique, which measures the rate of carbon monoxide uptake during a 10-second breath hold and uses alveolar volume calculated from helium dilution during the single-breath test. This will underestimate alveolar volume in patients with severe COPD.

Arterial blood gases and oximetry. In advanced COPD, measurement of arterial blood gases is important to assess the degree of hypoxemia and hypercapnia and, particularly in exacerbations, to define the partial pressure of carbon dioxide in arterial blood ($PaCO_2$) and the pH.

Patients with an FEV_1 of less than 50% of the predicted value, or with clinical signs suggestive of respiratory failure, right heart failure or cor pulmonale, should be assessed with pulse oximetry to determine oxygen saturation. Blood gases should be assessed in those with oxygen saturation less than 92% while breathing air.

Recording the inspired oxygen concentration is essential when reporting blood gases, but it is also important to note that it may take at least 30 minutes for a change in inspired oxygen concentration to have a full effect on the partial pressure of oxygen in arterial blood (PaO_2), because equilibration of alveolar gas takes a long time in COPD.

Blood for measurement of blood gases should be obtained by arterial puncture. Respiratory failure is indicated by a PaO_2 below 8 kPa (60 mmHg) with or without a $PaCO_2$ above 6.7 kPa (50 mmHg) while breathing air. Finger or ear oximeters for assessing oxygenation (percentage oxygen saturation of arterial blood, SaO_2) are less reliable but, because of their ease of use, are commonly used in clinical practice. An SaO_2 of 88% or below indicates the need for supplemental oxygen. Oximeters can also be used to measure changes in oxygenation during acute exacerbations. However, oximeters cannot completely replace assessment of blood gas values, because measurements of $PaCO_2$ are often required.

The acid–base consequences of increases in $PaCO_2$ can be compensated for by renal conservation of bicarbonate, which is a relatively slow process. Acid–base status, particularly in mixed respiratory and metabolic disturbances, can be characterized by plotting values on an acid–base diagram (Figure 4.8). It can also be assessed from the arterial pH and bicarbonate.

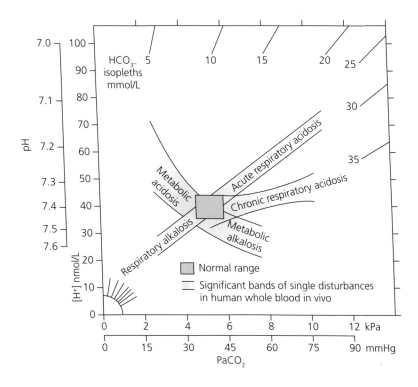

Figure 4.8 A non-logarithmic acid–base diagram derived from the measured acid–base status of patients within the five abnormal bands illustrated and of normal subjects (blue box). This plot of $PaCO_2$ against pH allows the likely acid–base disturbance and calculated bicarbonate value (obtained from the relevant isopleth) to be rapidly determined. Changes during treatment can be plotted serially for each patient. Reprinted from *The Lancet*. Flenley DC. Another r logarithmic acid–base diagram? *Lancet* 1971;1:961–5, © 1971 with p from Elsevier. HCO3., bicarbonate; $PaCO_2$, partial pressure of carbo arterial blood.

Exercise tests. Exercise induces an increase in oxygen consumption and carbon dioxide production in skeletal muscle. Patients with COPD have the same oxygen consumption for a given workload as normal individuals. However, their dead-space ventilation is higher, so a larger minute ventilation is needed to maintain carbon dioxide at a constant level. In many patients with COPD, expiratory airflow is limited within the tidal volume range. The only way to increase minute ventilation is to increase inspiratory flow or shift the end-expiratory position. Both of these maneuvers are problematic in patients with COPD and require more work from already compromised inspiratory muscles, or result in progressive overinflation, which increases both the work of breathing and symptoms. In addition, increased cardiac output with exercise can lead to increased perfusion of poorly ventilated areas. As a result of this ventilation–perfusion mismatch, arterial oxygenation can decline with exercise, in contrast to the improvement in oxygenation that is noted in normal individuals. Decline in oxygenation with exercise is generally monitored by measurement of percutaneous oxygen saturation. Exercise-induced desaturation can be an indication for supplemental oxygen therapy.

Three principal forms of exercise test are performed in COPD: progressive symptom-limited exercise, self-paced exercise and steady-state exercise. Other tests may be used in special circumstances.

Progressive symptom-limited exercise tests require patients to maintain exercise on a treadmill or a cycle until symptoms prevent them from continuing. The usual criteria for defining a maximum test are a heart rate greater than 85% of the predicted value or ventilation greater than 90% of the predicted value. The results are useful, particularly when simultaneous ECG and blood pressure monitoring are performed to assess whether coexisting cardiac or psychological factors contribute to exercise limitation.

Self-paced exercise tests are easy to perform and give information on more sustained exercise, which may be more relevant to performance in daily life. The 6-minute walk is the most commonly used test, with a coefficient of variation of around 8%. There may, however, be a learning effect that influences the result of repeated tests. This test is only useful in patients with moderately severe COPD ($FEV_1 < 1.5$ liters) who would be expected to have an exercise tolerance of less than 600 meters in 6 minutes. There is only a weak relationship between walking distance and FEV_1. A change in 30 meters over the 6-minute test may indicate a significant change in clinical status. Post-exercise pulse (the recovery of the pulse rate 1 minute after the test stops) also provides important information about the patient's functional status.

The shuttle walking test is an alternative in which the patient performs a paced walk between two points 10 meters apart (a shuttle). The pace of the walk is increased at regular intervals, dictated by bleeps on a tape recording, until the patient is forced to stop because of breathlessness. The number of completed shuttles is recorded.

Steady-state exercise tests require exercise at a sustainable percentage of maximum capacity for 3–6 minutes while blood gases are measured, enabling calculation of the dead space:tidal volume ratio and the passage through the lungs without oxygenation (shunt). This assessment is seldom required in patients with COPD.

Other more complex tests, such as assessing the lung pressure–volume curve, are difficult to undertake, because they require measurement of esophageal pressure with an esophageal balloon, and are not part of the routine assessment, but may be necessary in special circumstances. Measurements of small airway function, such as the nitrogen washout test, helium and air flow–volume loops and frequency dependency of compliance (the dependence of lung compliance on respiratory frequency), have poor reproducibility in patients with COPD. Although they can differentiate smokers from non-smokers, they are not useful in predicting which smokers will develop COPD and thus are not used in routine practice.

Additional pulmonary function tests, such as inspiratory capacity and lung volumes, are not usually required in routine assessment, but can provide further information. They are useful in some cases in which the diagnosis is uncertain and in assessing patients for surgery.

Assessment of breathlessness

Improvement in symptoms, particularly breathlessness, is one of the important goals of treatment in COPD. Although breathlessness is a subjective feature, it should be quantified. Several scales are available for assessing breathlessness objectively (see Chapter 3).

The modified Medical Research Council (mMRC) dyspnea scale (see Table 3.2) allows patients to rate their breathlessness according to t'

10 cm

Brisk walking uphill

Medium walking uphill

Brisk walking on level

Slow walking uphill   Heavy shopping

Medium walking on level

Light shopping

Bed-making

Slow walking on level   Washing yourself

Sitting

Sleeping

0 cm

Figure 4.9 Oxygen-cost diagram used in the assessment of breathlessness. The patient places a mark on the line to indicate when breathlessness occurs. The distance in centimeters from the zero point can be used to obtain a score.

activity that induces it. It is graded from 0 to 4 and is easy to use, but it is insensitive to change and may be more valuable as a baseline assessment than as a means of measuring the effect of treatment.

The oxygen-cost diagram is more sensitive to change than the mMRC dyspnea scale. It allows the patient to place a mark on a 10-cm line to represent the point beyond which breathlessness occurs (Figure 4.9).

Other scales allow quantification of breathlessness according to the intensity of the sensation. The Borg scale (see Table 3.1) is useful for measuring short-term changes in the intensity of breathlessness during a particular task. It is sensitive and reproducible. A simple analog scale is another method of allowing patients to rate the intensity of their breathlessness. As with the oxygen-cost diagram, a 10-cm line is drawn on a page and the patient then marks on the line how intense their breathlessness is, from 'not at all' (0 cm) to 'intensely breathless' (10 cm). The score is the distance along the line that the patient has marked.

Health status

Health status, sometimes termed quality of life, is a measure of the impact of a disease on daily life and well-being. COPD has a marked effect on health status, particularly owing to the limitations posed by breathlessness on exercise, daily activities and social activities, as well as the reductions in expectations, mood and well-being that it causes. Several questionnaires are available for the measurement of health status, but they are mainly used in hospital rehabilitation programs and in research, and are not yet employed in clinical practice.

The Chronic Respiratory Disease Index Questionnaire is sensitive to change, but is very time-consuming and requires training to administer properly. The St George's Respiratory Questionnaire (SGRQ) is a self-completed questionnaire with three components that give a total score of overall health status: symptoms, measuring distress due to respiratory symptoms; activity, measuring disturbance of daily activities; and impact, measuring psychosocial function. The Breathing Problems Questionnaire is a similar self-completed questionnaire, which is easy to complete, but relatively insensitive to change. The SGRQ has been most validated in COPD. Although there is a relationship between the SGRQ and the FEV_1 as a percentage of the predicted value, the relationship is rather poor. It is clear from various studies that treatment-related improvement in the SGRQ health status can occur without any improvement in FEV_1. The threshold of clinical improvement is a change of four units in the SGRQ.

Exacerbations of COPD have a clear detrimental effect on health status.

The COPD Assessment Test (CAT) was developed using rigorous psychometric methods to measure health status. The CAT is an eight-item unidimensional measure of health status that correlates well with the SGRQ. The CAT score varies between 0 and 40. It worsens during exacerbations. The test is copyrighted, but is free for clinicians to use (www.catestonline.org).

Respiratory muscle function

Respiratory muscle function can be assessed by measuring maximum inspiratory and expiratory mouth pressure. These measurements can be useful in evaluating patients with breathlessness or exercise intolerance that is unexplained by the severity of the lung function abnormality, as well as patients with suspected peripheral muscle weakness.

Sleep studies

Patients with COPD become increasingly hypoxemic during sleep, particularly during rapid eye movement sleep. There is no evidence that measurement of nocturnal hypoxemia provides any further prognostic or clinically useful information in the assessment of patients with COPD unless coexisting sleep apnea syndrome is suspected. Individuals who desaturate during the night may, however, be candidates for oxygen therapy.

Other assessments

Polycythemia. In patients with severe COPD, identifying polycythemia is important since it predisposes to vascular events. Polycythemia should be suspected when the hematocrit is more than 47% in women and more than 52% in men, and/or the hemoglobin is greater than 9.9 mmol/L (16 g/dL) in women and greater than 11.2 mmol/L (18 g/dL) in men, provided other causes of spurious polycythemia due to decreased plasma volume, such as occurs with dehydration, can be excluded.

Anemia is now recognized to be more common than previously thought and may affect over 25% of patients with COPD. The presence of anemia indicates a poor prognosis in patients with COPD receiving long-term oxygen treatment.

Screening for α1-antitrypsin deficiency should be considered in all patients who develop COPD since α1-antitrypsin can present with any manifestation of the disease. Societies' specific screening guidelines differ, with some recommendations incorporating local prevalence of α1-antitrypsin deficiency. Serum concentrations of α1-antitrypsin below 15–20% of the normal value are highly suggestive of deficiency. These findings should lead to family screening and appropriate counseling and, where available, consideration for replacement therapy.

Electrocardiography. Routine ECG is not required in the assessment of patients with COPD, and is an insensitive technique in the diagnosis of cor pulmonale.

Pulmonary arterial pressure. Patients with chronic hypoxemia may have mild-to-moderate pulmonary hypertension (mean pulmonary arterial pressure 30–45 mmHg). Measurement of pulmonary arterial pressure is not routinely recommended in clinical practice as it does not add any further information beyond that obtained by assessing arterial blood gases.

Differential diagnosis

It is often difficult to differentiate some patients with chronic asthma from those with COPD, and it is often assumed that asthma and COPD coexist in these patients. Other conditions to be considered in the differential diagnosis of COPD are listed in Table 4.5.

TABLE 4.5

Features of COPD and other conditions to be considered in the differential diagnosis

COPD
- Onset in midlife
- Slowly progressive symptoms
- Exposure to risk factors (e.g. tobacco smoking, occupational dust)
- Breathlessness during exercise
- Largely irreversible airflow limitation

Asthma
- Onset in early life
- Variable symptoms
- Particularly variable at night or the early morning
- Associated features of atopy, allergy, rhinitis and eczema
- Family history of atopy/asthma
- Largely reversible airflow limitation

Tuberculosis
- Chest radiograph shows lung infiltrate
- Onset at all ages
- Microbiological confirmation
- High local prevalence of tuberculosis

Bronchiectasis
- Large volumes of purulent sputum
- Associated bacterial infection
- Clubbing
- Coarse crackles on auscultation
- Bronchial wall thickening and bronchial dilatation seen on chest radiograph or CT scan

Congestive cardiac failure
- Presence of fine basal crackles on auscultation
- Dilated heart and evidence of pulmonary edema on chest radiograph
- Lung function tests indicate restrictive defect (see Figure 4.3)

Obliterative bronchiolitis
- Onset at a younger age
- Non-smokers affected
- May have history of rheumatoid arthritis or fume exposure
- Mosaic pattern on expiratory CT scan

CT, computed tomography.

Key points – lung function tests

- Spirometry is the most important measurement in COPD and is essential for diagnosis. Forced expiratory volume in 1 second (FEV_1) and forced vital capacity (FVC) are recorded in absolute values (liters) and also as a percentage of the predicted values for the individual depending on age, height, sex and ethnic origin.
- An FEV_1 over 80% of the predicted value is considered to be normal. This does not exclude the presence of disease.
- A post-bronchodilator FEV_1:FVC ratio below 0.7 indicates chronic airflow limitation and is a diagnostic criterion for COPD.
- A standardized technique must be employed in spirometry assessment. It is critical that the expiratory flow trace reaches a plateau to prove that the patient has reached the FVC.
- Reversibility testing to bronchodilators is useful in differential diagnosis to distinguish those with marked reversibility indicative of asthma.
- There is no standard assessment of reversibility; generally, however, an improvement in FEV_1 of both 200 mL and 12% over the baseline is interpreted as a positive result.
- Peak expiratory flow rate is not the best assessment of airway obstruction in COPD and may underestimate the degree of airway obstruction.
- Further tests of lung volumes and the diffusing capacity in the lung for carbon monoxide may be helpful in some cases.

Key references

Borg G. Psychophysical basis of perceived exertion. *Med Sci Sports Exerc* 1982;84:377–81.

COPD Assessment Test. www.catestonline.org, last accessed 19 January 2016.

Gibson GJ, MacNee W. Chronic obstructive pulmonary disease: investigations and assessment of severity. *Eur Respir Mon* 2006;38:24–40.

Global Initiative for Chronic Obstructive Lung Disease (GOLD). *Global Strategy for the Diagnosis, Management, and Prevention of Chronic Obstructive Pulmonary Disease*. Updated December 2015. www.goldcopd.org/uploads/users/files/GOLD_Report%202016.pdf, last accessed 19 January 2016.

Guyatt GH, Berman LB, Townsend M et al. A measure of quality of life for clinical trials in chronic lung disease. *Thorax* 1987;42:773–8.

Jones, PW, Harding G, Berry P et al. Development and first validation of the COPD Assessment Test. *Eur Respir J* 2009;34: 648–54.

Jones PW, Quirk FH, Baveystock CM, Littlejohns P. A self-complete measure for chronic airflow limitation: the St. George's questionnaire. *Am Rev Respir Dis* 1992;147:832–8.

McGavin CR, Artvinli M, Naoe H. Dyspnoea, disability and distance walked: a comparison of estimates of exercise performance in respiratory disease. *BMJ* 1978;2:241–3.

Noseda A, Carpeiaux JP, Schmerber J. Dyspnoea assessed by visual analogue scale in patients with obstructive lung disease during progressive and high intensity exercise. *Thorax* 1992;47:363–8.

Rennard S, Thomashow B, Crapo J et al. Introducing the COPD Foundation Guide for Diagnosis and Management of COPD, recommendations of the COPD Foundation. *COPD* 2013;10: 378–89.

Rodriguez-Roisin R, MacNee W. Pathophysiology of chronic obstructive pulmonary disease. *Eur Respir Mon* 2006;38:177–200.

Singh SJ, Morgan MDL, Scott SC et al. The development of the shuttle walking test of disability in patients with chronic airway obstruction. *Thorax* 1992;47:1019–24.

No features specific for COPD are seen on a plain posterior–anterior chest radiograph. The features usually described are those of severe emphysema. However, there may be no abnormalities, even in patients with very appreciable disability. Recent improvements in imaging techniques, particularly the advent of CT and, more recently, high-resolution CT (HRCT), have provided more sensitive means of diagnosing emphysema in life.

Plain chest radiography

The most reliable radiographic signs of emphysema can be classified by their causes of overinflation, vascular changes and bullae.

Overinflation of the lungs results in the following radiographic features:
- a low flattened diaphragm (Figure 5.1): the diaphragm is abnormally low if the border of the diaphragm in the midclavicular line is at or below the anterior end of the seventh rib; and the diaphragm is flattened if the perpendicular height from a line drawn between the costal and cardiophrenic angles to the border of the diaphragm is less than 1.5 cm
- increased retrosternal airspace, visible on the lateral film at a point 3 cm below the manubrium when the horizontal distance from the posterior surface of the aorta to the sternum exceeds 4.5 cm
- an obtuse costophrenic angle on the posterior–anterior or lateral chest radiograph
- an inferior margin of the retrosternal airspace 3 cm or less from the anterior aspect of the diaphragm.

Vascular changes associated with emphysema result from loss of alveolar walls and are shown on the plain chest radiograph by:
- a reduction in the size and number of pulmonary vessels, particularly at the periphery of the lung
- vessel distortion, producing increased branching angles, excess straightening or bowing of vessels
- areas of transradiancy.

Figure 5.1 Plain chest radiographs of generalized emphysema particularly affecting the lower zones. (a) Posterior–anterior radiograph showing a low, flat diaphragm (below the anterior ends of the seventh ribs), obtuse costophrenic angles and reduced vessel markings in lower zones, which are transradiant. (b) Lateral radiograph showing a low, flat and inverted diaphragm and widened retrosternal transradiancy (white arrows) that approaches the diaphragm inferiorly (blue arrows).

Assessment of the vascular loss in emphysema clearly depends on the quality of the radiograph. A generally increased transradiancy may simply be due to overexposure.

The development of right ventricular hypertrophy produces non-specific cardiac enlargement on the plain chest radiograph. Pulmonary hypertension may be suggested, taking measurements from the plain chest radiograph of the width of the right descending pulmonary artery, just below the right hilum, where the borders of the artery are delineated against the air in the lungs laterally and the right main-stem bronchus medially. The upper limit of the normal range of the width of the artery in this area is 16 mm in men and 15 mm in women. This increase in pulmonary artery size is often associated with a rapid diminution in the size of the vessels as they branch into the pulmonary periphery. Although these measurements can be used to detect the presence or absence of pulmonary hypertension, they cannot accurately predict the level of the pulmonary artery pressure and they are not felt to be particularly sensitive.

Bullae may be seen as focal areas of transradiancy surrounded by hairline walls.

Computed tomography

CT scanning has been used to detect and quantify emphysema. Techniques can be divided into those that use visual assessment of low-density areas on the CT scan, which can be either semiquantitative or quantitative, and those that use CT lung density to quantify areas of low X-ray attenuation. These two techniques are usually employed to measure macroscopic or microscopic emphysema, respectively. Use of inspiratory and expiratory phases during CT scanning helps to determine air-trapping and small airways disease.

Visual assessment of emphysema on CT scanning (Figure 5.2) reveals:
- areas of low attenuation without obvious margins or walls
- attenuation and pruning of the vascular tree
- abnormal vascular configurations.

The sign that correlates best with areas of macroscopic emphysema is an area of low attenuation. Visual inspection of the CT scan can locate areas of macroscopic emphysema, though a visual assessment of the extent of macroscopic emphysema is insensitive and subjective with high intra- and inter-observer variability.

It is possible to distinguish the various types of emphysema using HRCT, particularly when the changes are not severe. The distinction depends on the distribution of the lesions: those of centrilobular emphysema are patchy and prominent in the upper zones; whereas those of panlobular emphysema are diffuse throughout the lung zones (see Figure 5.2). It is generally acceptable to select patients with upper lung zone emphysema for volume reduction surgery by visual inspection of an HRCT by an experienced radiologist and surgeon.

Measurement of lung density on CT in terms of Hounsfield units (a scale of X-ray attenuation where bone is +1000 Hounsfield units, water is 0 Hounsfield units and air is –1000 Hounsfield units) provides a more quantitative way of assessing emphysema (Figure 5.3), particularly at the microscopic level.

Figure 5.2 High-resolution CT scans of the lungs. (a) Diffuse panlobular emphysema. (b) More patchy centrilobular emphysema with bullae.

A quantitative approach to assessing macroscopic emphysema has been taken by highlighting picture elements, or pixels, within the lung fields in a predetermined low density range, between –910 and –1000 Hounsfield units (the most widely accepted threshold is –950 Hounsfield units), which is known as the 'density mask' technique.

If CT scanning is to be used to measure microscopic emphysema, care should be taken to standardize the scanning conditions, particularly the lung volume, and to calibrate the CT scanner, since these factors affect CT lung density. Patient factors (e.g. obesity) can also affect quantification of emphysema on CT; in such cases, patients can be asked to inhale to a certain lung volume using respiratory-gated CT.

These techniques have not, as yet, been sufficiently standardized for use in clinical practice, but density measurements have been shown to correlate with morphometric measurements of distal airspace size in resected lungs. Assessment of CT lung density is currently being used in clinical trials to demonstrate progressive emphysema.

Detection of bullae. Whether a bulla is detected on a chest radiograph depends on its size and the degree to which it is obscured by overlying lung. CT scanning is much more sensitive than plain chest radiography in detecting bullae and can be used to determine their number, size and position.

Other features can be assessed on the CT scan including bone density, coronary artery calcification and pulmonary artery size.

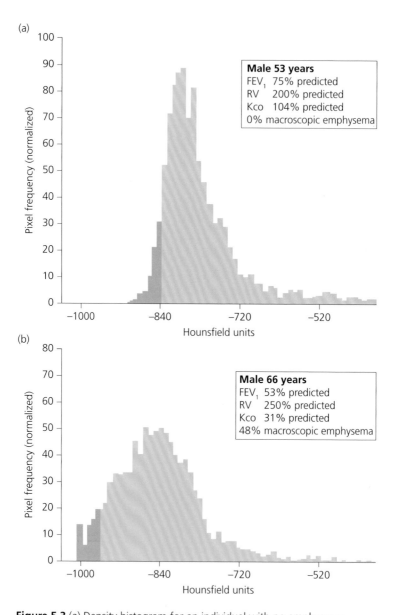

Figure 5.3 (a) Density histogram for an individual with no emphysema.
(b) Density histogram for a patient with severe emphysema. The darker area
represents the lowest 5% of the distribution. FEV_1, forced expiratory volume in
1 second; Kco, carbon monoxide transfer coefficient; RV, residual volume.

Echocardiography

Echocardiography has been used to assess the right ventricle and to detect pulmonary hypertension in COPD. However, overinflation of the chest increases the retrosternal airspace, which then transmits sound waves poorly, making echocardiography difficult in patients with COPD. Nevertheless, an adequate examination can be achieved in 65–85% of patients with COPD.

Two-dimensional echocardiography has been used in the investigation of right ventricular dimensions and is superior to clinical methods since it shows reasonable correlations between pulmonary artery pressure and various right ventricular dimensions.

Pulsed-wave Doppler echocardiography has been used to assess the ejection flow dynamics of the right ventricle in patients with pulmonary hypertension. The parameters measured include: acceleration time (in milliseconds), which is defined as the time between the onset of ejection to peak velocity; right ventricular pre-ejection time (in milliseconds), which is the interval from the Q wave of the ECG to the beginning of the forward flow; and right ventricular ejection time (in milliseconds), which is the interval between the onset and termination of flow in the right ventricular outflow tract. Although the pulsed-wave Doppler technique is useful in differentiating patients with an elevated pulmonary arterial pressure from those with normal pulmonary arterial pressure, it is not as accurate as the continuous-wave Doppler technique in assessing pulmonary arterial pressure.

Continuous-wave Doppler echocardiography is the best technique for non-invasive evaluation of pulmonary arterial pressure; the tricuspid gradient assessed in this way can be used to calculate the right ventricular systolic pressure. The technique estimates the pressure gradient across the regurgitant jet recorded by Doppler ultrasound. The maximum velocity of the regurgitant jet is measured from the continuous-wave Doppler recordings, and the simplified Bernoulli equation is used to calculate the maximum pressure gradient between the right ventricle and the right atrium as:

$P_{RV} - P_{RA} = 4v^2$

where P_{RV} and P_{RA} are the right ventricular and right atrial pressures and v is the maximum velocity.

The right atrial pressure is estimated from clinical examination of the jugular venous pressure. There is still debate as to whether this technique is sufficiently sensitive and reproducible to monitor longitudinal changes in pulmonary arterial pressure and the effects of therapeutic interventions, particularly in patients with COPD.

Other imaging modalities

Radionuclide-based ventilation/perfusion scanning can be used to assess regional lung function. This may be helpful in assessing predicted lung function after surgical resection and, therefore, patient selection for surgical resection, e.g. of a localized lung cancer, if significant COPD is present.

Key points – imaging

- No features on plain chest radiography are specific for COPD. The features usually described are those of severe emphysema, but no abnormality may be visible, even in patients with marked disability.
- CT scans can be used to quantify emphysema, either by visual assessment of high-resolution scanning or by CT lung density measurements.
- CT scanning is the best way to detect and assess bullous disease.
- CT scanning is the standard way to assess patients for volume reduction surgery.
- Echocardiography, particularly continuous-wave Doppler echocardiography, can be used to assess pulmonary arterial pressure in patients with COPD.

Key references

Coxson HO, Rogers RM. New concepts in the radiological concepts of COPD. *Semin Respir Crit Care Med* 2005;26:211–20.

Freidman PJ. Imaging studies in emphysema. *Proc Am Thorac Soc* 2008;5:494–500.

O'Brien C, Guest PJ, Hill SL, Stockley RA. Physiological and radiological characterization of patients diagnosed with chronic obstructive pulmonary disease in primary care. *Thorax* 2000;55: 635–42.

Cigarette smoking is the single most important factor in the development of COPD. Smoking cessation is therefore the single most important therapeutic intervention. The earlier a smoker quits, the more advantages accrue.

Most cigarette smokers (> 85%) are addicted to nicotine and experience a well-defined withdrawal syndrome to varying degrees following cessation (Table 6.1). These symptoms peak in the first few days following cessation and gradually decrease after 2–3 weeks. Episodes of craving, which may be intense, may recur for many years; they are often initiated by environmental or behavioral cues associated with smoking. It is important that smokers are informed that these cravings will subside with or without relapse to smoking.

Smoking should not be oversimplified as merely a lifestyle choice, but, owing to the addiction, should be considered as a primary disease entity in itself. In this context, smoking is properly classified as a chronic, often

TABLE 6.1

Withdrawal syndrome following smoking cessation*

- Dysphoric or depressed mood
- Insomnia
- Irritability, frustration or anger
- Anxiety
- Difficulty concentrating
- Restlessness
- Decreased heart rate
- Increased appetite or weight gain
- Craving to smoke[†]

*Defined in the *Diagnostic and Statistical Manual of Mental Disorders*. 4th edn. Arlington, Virginia: American Psychiatric Association, 2000.
[†]Not included in the *Diagnostic and Statistical Manual of Mental Disorders* for 'logical reasons', but a characteristic of the syndrome.

relapsing, disease. Smoking cessation is thus not simply a matter of personal choice, but is a legitimate therapeutic intervention, the goal of which is to induce a 'remission' in smoking.

There is evidence that smokers differ in their biological propensity to become smokers and that genetic factors may affect their ability to quit. Therapeutic interventions targeted at individual smokers' susceptibilities are under intensive investigation. Available therapies can nevertheless help a substantial minority of smokers to quit.

Among adult smokers, approximately 70% wish to stop smoking, and as many as 45% make a serious attempt in each year. Despite this, only 2% of smokers successfully quit spontaneously in a year. Simple physician advice to quit can increase these rates to 5–6%. Additional non-pharmacological support, which can include behavioral, cognitive and motivational support, and pharmacological therapy can further increase quit rates. Current recommendations are, therefore, that all physicians establish smoking status as a 'vital sign' at every visit and undertake appropriate smoking cessation intervention (Figure 6.1). These steps ensure that smokers receive maximum encouragement to quit.

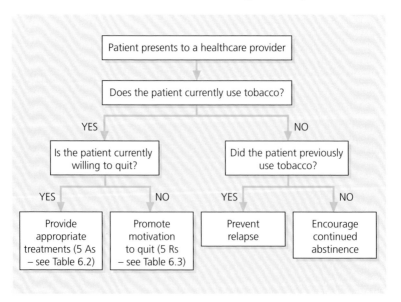

Figure 6.1 Brief anti-smoking intervention to be undertaken at every visit to the healthcare provider.

- Brief interventions should be implemented in all practices.
- Intensive interventions are appropriate for many patients with COPD. Each practitioner caring for patients with COPD should have the option of referring patients for intensive intervention.
- System approaches ensure smoking cessation intervention is integrated into each practice and is fully supported by the healthcare system.

Brief interventions

Brief interventions can be highly effective for many smokers. The five As (Table 6.2) provide key steps for a brief intervention that can be accomplished within a few minutes and can be tailored to the needs of each smoker.

Smokers not yet ready to quit should be provided with a brief intervention to increase motivation. This should be sympathetic and non-confrontational, and should provide patient-specific information. The five Rs can provide guidance in this respect (Table 6.3). The patient should also understand that the physician is working in their best interest and will

TABLE 6.2

The five As for physician intervention

Ask
Implement a system that ensures that tobacco use is queried and documented for every patient at every clinic visit

Advise
In a clear, strong and personalized manner, urge all tobacco users to quit

Assess
Ask every tobacco user if he or she is willing to attempt to quit at this time (e.g. within the next 30 days)

Assist
Help the patient make a quit plan, provide practical counseling and intra-treatment social support, help the patient obtain extra-treatment social support, recommend use of approved pharmacotherapy (except in special circumstances) and provide supplementary materials

Arrange
Schedule follow-up contact, either in person or by telephone

TABLE 6.3

The five Rs for smoker motivation

Relevance
- Personalize the reasons to quit. This may include issues in addition to COPD

Risks
- Acute: dyspnea, cough, exacerbations, increased carbon monoxide levels
- Chronic: COPD progression, cancer, cardiovascular disease, osteoporosis, peptic ulcer
- Environmental: disease risk to spouse and other household members, increased risk of smoking and of disease in children

Rewards
- Improves health
- Improves self-image, sense of taste and smell
- Saves money
- Sets a good example for children

Roadblocks
- Withdrawal symptoms
- Fear of failure
- Weight gain
- Lack of support
- Depression
- Enjoyment of tobacco

Repetition
- Most smokers make several quit attempts before achieving long-term abstinence; smoking can be regarded as a chronic relapsing condition, but prolonged remissions are possible

be prepared to offer appropriate smoking cessation counseling when the patient is ready.

Every smoker ready to attempt to quit should be offered the highest probability of success. Non-pharmacological support, pharmacological treatment and follow-up all contribute to success.

Behavioral support. Data show clearly that the more behavioral support offered the more likely a smoker is to quit. Many smokers, however, will not attend intensive behavioral programs. Brief behavioral help is therefore appropriate for most individuals and a number of approaches are shown in Table 6.4. The efficacy of widely available telephone quit lines has been well demonstrated. In addition, some studies have suggested efficacy for the many internet-based interventions that have been developed. However, many of these do not have supporting evidence.

Pharmacological treatment. All smokers making a serious attempt to quit should be offered pharmacological treatment (in the absence of contraindications). Treatment with first-line medicines for smoking

TABLE 6.4

Behavioral support for smokers trying to quit

Help establish a quit plan
- Set a quit date (ideally within 2 weeks)
- Tell family and friends
- Anticipate challenges
- Remove tobacco products

Counseling
- Be aware that abstinence is essential (most smokers who smoke at all after the quit date will relapse to the previous habit)
- Utilize experience from previous quit attempts
- Anticipate challenges
- Avoid alcohol (the most frequent relapses occur with concurrent alcohol)
- Consider the effect of other smokers in the household (supportive, obstructive, prepared to quit too?)

Encourage other support
- Enlist family, friends and coworkers to assist
- Find support groups

Provide educational materials
- Should be available in every clinician's office. Many are available through a variety of agencies

cessation can double or triple quit rates compared with those achieved without pharmacological support. Second-line treatments should be considered for smokers who have failed first-line treatment.

First-line treatments for smoking cessation include nicotine replacement therapy, varenicline and bupropion (also known as amfebutamone).

Nicotine replacement therapy is available in several formulations: polacrilex gum, transdermal systems, inhalers, nasal sprays and lozenges. Several other formulations are under investigation. All are similar in efficacy and approximately double quit rates compared with placebo, though they differ in clinical use. This form of therapy has been in use the longest and many over-the-counter formulations are available. Many patients will therefore have had prior experience with these treatments.

The use of nicotine replacement therapy for smoking cessation is based on the pharmacokinetics of nicotine as a psychoactive drug. The 'hit' associated with nicotine depends on both the amount of nicotine that reaches the brain and the rate of rise in the concentration. The peaks not only provide the psychoactive effect of nicotine, but also contribute to both the psychological and the biological reinforcing mechanisms leading to addiction. Withdrawal symptoms are believed to develop when nicotine levels fall below a certain threshold (Figure 6.2). This generally occurs several hours after the last cigarette, as nicotine has a half-life of the order of hours in most individuals. The concept behind nicotine replacement therapy, therefore, is to provide a steady-state level that can protect against the symptoms of withdrawal without providing the reinforcement that contributes to addiction.

Currently available nicotine formulations provide only partial nicotine replacement for most smokers, and none completely prevents withdrawal symptoms, but they do reduce them. More importantly, nicotine replacement therapies increase quit rates. The general strategy for their use is to establish a quit day and to start nicotine replacement on that day. Therapy is then continued for 10 weeks to 6 months. Individual preferences for the various formulations allow the physician some choice in individualizing therapy.

The various formulations also have different pharmacokinetics. This is likely to affect their potential to sustain addiction; many individuals have substituted nicotine gum for cigarettes, but remained addicted. It is

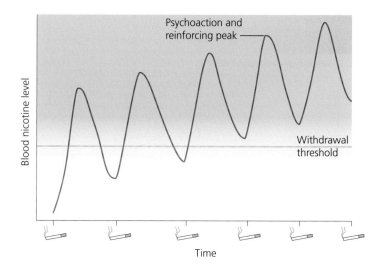

Figure 6.2 Peaks in blood nicotine level provide the psychoactive effect, and contribute to the psychological and biological reinforcing mechanisms leading to addiction. Withdrawal symptoms are believed to develop when the nicotine level falls below a certain threshold.

generally considered, however, that the health hazards associated with the gum are dramatically less than those associated with smoking.

Because the available formulations generally provide incomplete nicotine replacement, combination therapy can be considered. In particular, the use of a nicotine transdermal system (patch) in combination with another formulation that can provide as-needed nicotine during times of craving – a 'patch-plus' strategy – has been recommended. This use, while supported by several studies, is 'off-label'.

Varenicline functions as a partial agonist and is selective for the α4β2 nicotinic receptor. Consistent with its ability to partially activate this receptor, individuals who quit smoking while being treated with varenicline have reduced withdrawal symptoms. In addition, individuals who continue to smoke experience less of the rewarding effects of nicotine, consistent with the antagonism expected of a partial agonist (Figure 6.3). Clinical trials suggest that varenicline can achieve abstinence rates that are three times better than placebo, and that are better than both bupropion and nicotine replacement therapy.

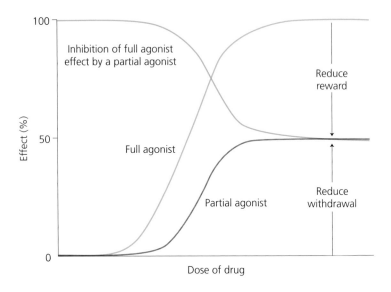

Figure 6.3 The actions of a partial agonist for smoking cessation. A full agonist (green line) results in increasing effect with increasing dose and resembles the effect of nicotine. A partial agonist (red line) results in a partial effect, no matter how much is added. By mimicking the effect of nicotine, varenicline may reduce the effects of withdrawal. In addition, a partial agonist blocks the full effect of a full agonist (blue line) and, in this way, varenicline may reduce the rewarding effects of nicotine.

Varenicline is usually started at a dose of 0.5 mg once daily for 3 days, increased to 0.5 mg twice daily for 3 days and then increased to 1 mg twice daily. The slow increase in dose reduces the incidence of nausea, which is the most common adverse effect. Other relatively common side effects include insomnia and abnormal dreams. Because the drug is primarily excreted unchanged by the kidney, no change in dose is required for concurrent hepatic disease, but a decrease in dose to 0.5 mg/day is recommended in patients with compromised renal function (e.g. creatinine clearance < 30 mL/minute).

Mood and behavioral disturbances have been reported in patients treated with varenicline, including depression, agitation, suicidal thoughts, and aggressive and erratic behavior. It may be difficult to separate some of these symptoms from nicotine withdrawal. The reports have, however, led to a labeling change in the USA, and patients, their families and caregivers should be alerted to monitor for these neuropsychiatric symptoms. Varenicline has also been associated with drowsiness, and the label contains a warning for users of heavy machinery. An early meta-analysis suggested increased cardiac risk with varenicline use, but that report, which was felt to be flawed, was not substantiated by a subsequent meta-analysis or additional study.

There are no data, as yet, regarding the combination of varenicline with other medications for smoking cessation.

Bupropion also acts directly on the CNS, and is in use as an antidepressant. It approximately doubles quit rates compared with placebo, and may be particularly effective in individuals with a history of depression. Bupropion and nicotine replacement therapy can be used in combination. Bupropion is generally started 1 week before the quit day so that adequate blood levels can be achieved. The usual initial dose is 150 mg once a day and is increased to twice a day after 3 days if tolerated.

Bupropion should not be used in individuals at risk of seizures or with a history of bulimia or anorexia, and should not be prescribed for patients who are currently receiving bupropion for the treatment of depression. It carries the same warning related to mood changes, depression and suicidality as varenicline.

Second-line therapies include clonidine and nortriptyline. Clonidine has been evaluated in several clinical trials and, though it is not approved and the individual trials did not consistently show statistically significant benefits, a meta-analysis supports its use. Physicians comfortable with this medication can consider it an aid to smoking cessation.

The antidepressant nortriptyline has also been evaluated in several clinical trials, which have shown clinical efficacy. This agent is available as an antidepressant and can therefore be used off-label for smoking cessation by physicians comfortable with its use.

Electronic cigarettes and other recreational nicotine products. A number of non-cigarette nicotine-containing products have been introduced as consumer products. In contrast to pharmaceutical nicotine replacement, the safety of these products is generally untested. There may be benefits for individual smokers who switch from cigarettes to such products, but this is not demonstrated. If such products discourage smokers from quitting, or encourage non-smokers to start using nicotine, which is addictive, they could have substantial adverse public health effects. Currently, no data have demonstrated the efficacy of electronic cigarettes as a smoking cessation aid. For this reason, smokers interested in combustible tobacco use cessation should be offered approved modalities (e.g. nicotine replacement therapy, nicotinic receptor agonists).

Follow-up evaluations. Success in smoking cessation is closely linked to follow-up. All smokers making a serious attempt to quit should therefore be offered follow-up assessment. Such assessments can deal with specific problems related to cessation and medication use, and can provide behavioral support. Follow-up 1–2 weeks after the quit day is generally recommended. Additional follow-ups can also be beneficial.

Intensive interventions

Intensive interventions are more elaborate than the brief interventions described above. Generally speaking, they require trained counselors and can be conducted either as individual or group sessions. Most often, multiple sessions are necessary. Only a minority of smokers referred for intensive programs will attend. Such programs can, however, provide important support for many smokers, and every practitioner should be able to refer patients for intensive intervention.

Approach to system integration

Cigarette smoking should be regarded as a primary disease, and its treatment should be integrated into each healthcare system. This should include adequate training of personnel to interview patients for smoking status as a 'vital sign'. The healthcare system should also provide adequate support for smoking cessation efforts and personnel at all levels should be active participants in smoking cessation interventions. Data show that quit rates increase when more personnel at more levels participate in smoking cessation therapy.

For more detailed information, see *Fast Facts: Smoking Cessation.*

Key points – smoking cessation

- Smoking should be regarded as a primary chronic relapsing disease.
- All serious attempts to quit should be maximally supported with behavioral and pharmacological interventions.
- Repeated efforts by the physician are required to provide sufficient motivation for a quit attempt.
- Relapses are common, and should engender repeated attempts.
- Smoking cessation activities should be an integrated part of every medical practice.

Key references

Daughton D, Susman J, Sitorius M et al. Transdermal nicotine therapy and primary care. Importance of counseling, demographic and patient selection factors on one-year quit rates. The Nebraska Primary Practice Smoking Cessation Trial Group. *Arch Fam Med* 1998;7: 425–30.

Drummond MB, Upson D. Electronic cigarettes. Potential harms and benefits. *Ann Am Thorac Soc* 2014;11:236–42.

Fiore MC, Panel Chair. *Clinical Practice Guideline. Treating Tobacco Use and Dependence: 2008 Update.* www.bphc.hrsa.gov/buckets/ treatingtobacco.pdf, last accessed 19 January 2016.

Fiore MC. US public health service clinical practice guideline: treating tobacco use and dependence. *Respir Care* 2000;45:1200–62.

Fiore MC, Bailey WC, Cohen SJ. *Smoking cessation.* Guideline technical report no. 18. Rockville, MD: US Dept of Health and Human Services, Public Health Service, Agency for Health Care Policy and Research. Publication No. AHCPR 97-No4, October 1997.

Rennard SI, Hepp L. Cigarette smoke induced disease. In: Stockley R, Rennard S, Rabe K, Celli B, eds. *Chronic Obstructive Pulmonary Disease.* Oxford: Wiley–Blackwell, 2006.

Schwartz JL. Review and evaluation of smoking cessation methods: the United States and Canada, 1978–1985. NIH Publication No. 87-2940, 1987:1125–56.

West R, Shiffman S. *Fast Facts: Smoking Cessation,* 3rd edn. Oxford: Health Press Limited, 2016.

Overall strategy

The COPD Foundation Guide recommends basing clinical management on the assessment of seven domains (see Table 3.4). Several of the medications and treatment options address multiple domains (Table 7.1).

The treatment strategy for stable COPD recommended by the Global initiative for chronic Obstructive Lung Disease (GOLD) considers patient symptoms and future risk of exacerbations (see Figure 3.2; Table 7.2).

Pharmacological treatment: bronchodilators

Rationale and physiology of benefit. Bronchodilators are the first-line treatment for patients with COPD. It may seem paradoxical that COPD, which by definition has, at best, limited reversibility, is treated with bronchodilators as first-line therapy. However, even small improvements in airflow can make a significant difference to patients with COPD.

Most people have some degree of airway smooth muscle tone, including patients with COPD. Thus, normal individuals will often experience a very modest improvement in airflow when given a bronchodilator. Sedentary normal individuals seldom notice any ease in breathing as a result. Patients with COPD, however, for whom the cost of breathing is substantially greater, especially on exercising, often notice significant improvements in the ease with which they breathe with even modest improvements in airflow.

Even in the absence of measurable improvements in airflow, patients with COPD may still derive benefit from bronchodilators. The likely explanation is that airflow in patients with COPD is not only compromised but is irregularly compromised. As a result, the rate at which different portions of the lung empty during exhalation is variable. With increasing respiratory rate, the areas most severely affected become hyperinflated (see Chapter 2). Subtle improvements in airflow, which result in better matching of the rates with which various portions of the lung empty, probably have an important effect on lung volumes, particularly with increasing respiratory rates, even if total airflow is relatively unaffected. This can

TABLE 7.1

Treatment options for stable COPD based on COPD Foundation severity domains

		Therapy						
	SABA	LAMA, LABA or LAMA+LABA	ICS/LABA	PDE4 inhibitor	Oxygen	Exercise; rehabilitation	Lung volume reduction surgery	Azithromycin
Clinical domain								
SG-1	First line, prn	Possibly						
SG-2/3	First line, prn	First line	Yes	Yes*				
Regular symptoms	First line, prn	First line	Yes			First line		
Exacerbation risk high		First line	First line	Yes*				Yes
Oxygenation								
– at rest					Yes			
– episodic					Possibly			
Emphysema							Selected cases	
Chronic bronchitis				Yes*				
Comorbidities								

*All three severity domains (regular symptoms, high exacerbation risk, chronic bronchitis) must be present.
ICS, inhaled corticosteroid; LABA, long-acting β₂ agonist; LAMA, long-acting antimuscarinic; PDE4, phosphodiesterase 4 inhibitor; prn, as needed; SABA, short-acting β₂ agonist; SG-1, spirometry grade 1 – mild COPD (see Figure 4.4); SG-2/3, spirometry grade 2/3 – moderate to severe COPD (see Figure 4.4). Source: COPD Foundation Guide. http://pocketconsultantguide.copdfoundation.org, last accessed 19 January 2016.

TABLE 7.2

GOLD guidelines for pharmacological therapy for stable COPD

Severity of COPD	First choice	Alternate choice	Other options
A	SABA; SAMA	LAMA; LABA; SAMA+SABA	Theophylline
B	LAMA; LABA	LAMA+LABA	SABA+/orSAMA; theophylline
C	ICS+LABA; LAMA	LAMA+LABA; LAMA+PDE4i; LABA+PDE4i	SABA+/orSAMA; theophylline
D	ICS+LABA+/or LAMA	ICS+LABA+LAMA; ICS+LABA+PDE4i; LAMA+LABA; LAMA+PDE4i	Carbocisteine (carbocysteine); SABA+/orSAMA; theophylline

GOLD severity groups: A, low risk and fewer symptoms; B, low risk and more symptoms; C, high risk and fewer symptoms; D, high risk and more symptoms. See Figure 3.2 for more information on how these groups are determined.
ICS, inhaled corticosteroid; LABA, long-acting β_2 agonist; LAMA, long-acting antimuscarinic; PDE4i, phosphodiesterase 4 inhibitor; SABA, short-acting β_2 agonist; SAMA, short-acting antimuscarinic.

lead to a gratifying apparent paradox in which a patient has significant clinical improvement in dyspnea on exertion in the absence of any measurable improvement in forced expiratory volume in 1 second (FEV_1) at rest.

Mode of delivery. To minimize side effects, brochodilators are best given by inhalation rather than systemically. When given by inhalation it is important to ensure that there is effective delivery of the drug, which requires proper technique of inhaler use. Ensuring that each patient is able to use the inhaler that is prescribed is essential. Moreoever, inhaler technique can deteriorate with time, so repeated assessment and education is needed.

Dosage. Bronchodilators are given on either an as-needed basis or on a regular basis to prevent or reduce symptoms. Dose responses as assessed by the change in FEV_1 are relatively flat for all classes of bronchodilators, so dosing is not based on spirometric response. Increasing doses above those conventionally prescribed can increase toxicity.

Clinical monitoring. In view of the above, all patients with COPD should be treated initially and aggressively with bronchodilators to control symptoms. Their response should be monitored with objective measures of airflow and on the basis of clinical outcomes, such as symptoms and performance. Adequate assessment of clinical response may require exercise challenge. It is common for patients with COPD to restrict their level of activity progressively as the disease worsens. This reduces dyspnea, but at the cost of an increasingly sedentary existence. Treatment with bronchodilators alone is often insufficient to treat such patients. Usually, improvements in physiological function can benefit the patient only if the bronchodilator treatment is used together with an aggressive rehabilitation program (see pages 113–17). Thus, though bronchodilators form first-line therapy in COPD, for their use to be successful they must be integrated into an appropriate management plan, such as that suggested in the GOLD strategy document (see Table 7.2) or the COPD Foundation Guide (see Table 7.1).

Treatment strategy based on severity classification. The following is based on the COPD Foundation Guide, as it is a more comprehensive classification of spirometric values (see Figure 4.4) and as the cut-off points are based on clinical decision points.

In mild COPD ($FEV_1 \geq 60\%$ predicted), treatment is based on the presence of symptoms. If dyspnea is present, short-acting bronchodilators (SABAs) can be given on an as-needed basis. Since dyspnea is most likely to develop following exercise, it may be prudent to give bronchodilators before exertion in order to facilitate a greater level of activity rather than to administer them following exertion. Long-acting bronchodilators (LABAs) may help to maintain high levels of activity on a regular basis.

In moderate COPD ($30\% \leq FEV_1 < 60\%$), regular treatment with one or more bronchodilator is recommended. Individuals who do not spontaneously complain of dyspnea will most commonly have limited their activity as a means to avoid shortness of breath. Use of bronchodilators for these patients needs to be integrated into an exercise and rehabilitation program aimed at restoring activity levels. LABAs are appealing, as optimizing airflow for as long as possible throughout the day and night seems advantageous in maximizing performance ability. Inhaled glucocorticosteroids (ICS) can be considered. They are most likely to be of benefit as the disease worsens and exacerbation frequency increases.

Classes of bronchodilator. There are three main classes of bronchodilator:

- β-agonists
- anticholinergics
- theophylline.

Both short-acting and long-acting agents or formulations are available in all three classes.

β-*agonists* act as bronchodilators by acting on the β_2-subclass of β-agonist receptors in airway smooth muscle, thereby increasing cyclic adenosine monophosphate (cAMP) levels (Figure 7.1), which in turn decreases airway smooth muscle tone. β-agonists can act on β-receptors on other cell types as well (e.g. the heart). By relaxing vascular smooth muscle, they can increase blood flow to relatively poorly ventilated areas and may thus cause a reduction in oxygenation in some settings. Effects on airway epithelial cells and inflammatory cells may be beneficial (see below), but the clinical importance of all these non-bronchodilator effects remains uncertain.

A variety of β-agonists are available in a number of formulations (Table 7.3). They fall roughly into two classes: short-acting and long-acting. Most of the commonly used β-agonists are relatively selective for the β_2-receptor subtype. As a result, they have relatively fewer cardiac side effects than the older non-selective β-agonists such as isoprenaline (isoproterenol), as the most important β-receptors in the heart are β_1-receptors. However, because the heart has some β_2-receptors, no selective agent will be entirely free of cardiac effects.

Tremor can be troublesome in some older patients treated with higher doses of β_2-agonists. Higher doses of β_2-agonists can also cause hypokalemia, particularly when combined with diuretic therapy.

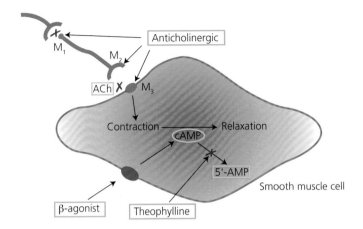

Figure 7.1 Mechanisms of action of bronchodilators: anticholinergics block muscarinic receptors so that acetylcholine (ACh) is unable to act upon them; β-agonists increase levels of cyclic adenosine monophosphate (cAMP); theophylline blocks conversion of cAMP to 5′-adenosine monophosphate (5′-AMP). M_1, M_2 and M_3 are three distinct types of muscarinic cholinergic receptors.

Short-acting β-agonists. Most SABAs have a relatively rapid onset of action, achieving measurable bronchodilation within 5 minutes and a maximal effect in about 30 minutes (Figure 7.2). These agents have been shown to improve FEV_1 and symptoms, but the effect generally wanes after 2 hours, and the often-stated 4-hour duration of action is somewhat optimistic. As a result, for regular use, these agents must be administered 4–6 times daily.

The most widely used agent is salbutamol (albuterol). It is available in a number of formulations in metered-dose inhalers and nebulized solutions. Administration via a nebulizer may be appropriate for patients with extremely limited airflows and for individuals who cannot coordinate the use of a metered-dose inhaler. Many patients seem to derive benefit from the ritual aspects of applying the nebulizer mask. In some countries, patients prefer nebulizer therapy because it is covered to a greater degree by their healthcare insurance than metered-dose inhaler formulations.

Salbutamol is a chiral molecule and most preparations are racemic (i.e. mixtures of the levo and dextro forms). Only the levo form interacts

97

TABLE 7.3

Common β-agonist bronchodilator formulations

Drug	Inhaler (µg)	Nebulizer solution	Oral (mg)	Injectable	Duration of action (hours)
Short-acting					
Fenoterol	100–200 MDI	1 mg/mL	0.05% (syrup)	–	4–6
Salbutamol (albuterol)	100–200 MDI and DPI	5 mg/mL	5 (pill); 0.024% (syrup)	0.1 and 0.5 mg/vial	4–6
Levosalbutamol (levalbuterol)	45 MDI	0.63, 1.25 mg in 3 mL	–	–	5–8
Terbutaline	400, 500 MDI	–	2.5, 5	0.2 and 0.25 mg/vial	4–6
Long-acting					
Formoterol	4.5–12 MDI and DPI	20 µg in 2 mL	–	–	≥ 12
Arformoterol	–	15 µg in 2 mL	–	–	≥ 12
Salmeterol	25–50 MDI and DPI	–	–	–	≥ 12
Indacaterol	75–300 DPI	–	–	–	24
Olodaterol	5 MDI	–	–	–	24

DPI, dry-powder inhaler; MDI, metered-dose inhaler.

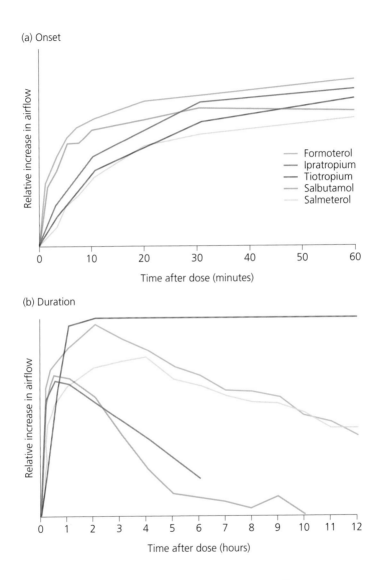

(a) Onset

Relative increase in airflow

— Formoterol
— Ipratropium
— Tiotropium
— Salbutamol
— Salmeterol

0   10   20   30   40   50   60

Time after dose (minutes)

(b) Duration

Relative increase in airflow

0 1 2 3 4 5 6 7 8 9 10 11 12

Time after dose (hours)

Figure 7.2 (a) Onset and (b) duration of action of bronchodilators.

with the β_2-receptor to have a beneficial effect, and it has been suggested that the dextro form contributes to the adverse effects. Preparations of the levo form alone, which may reduce adverse side effects, are available both as a metered-dose inhaler and as a nebulized solution.

β-agonists have a number of systemic side effects due to the total absorbed dose, including ventricular contractions, palpitations, tachycardia, tremor, sleep disturbances and hypokalemia. While topical deposition in the airway by inhalation increases the therapeutic index, a drug that is deposited in the mouth and swallowed can result in side effects without local benefit. Such side effects can be reduced by the use of spacers or other devices that decrease oral deposition of the drug.

Salbutamol can also be taken orally. As might be expected, oral administration results in a considerably higher systemic dose than the same dose delivered to the lungs by inhalation. As a result, the side effects of tachycardia and tremor are more common, so oral dosing is reserved for highly selected patients.

Slow-release oral formulations of salbutamol permit its use as a long-acting preparation, but do not alter the pharmacokinetics of the drug itself.

Long-acting β-agonists. Five LABAs are available for inhalation (see Table 7.3): formoterol (eformoterol), arformoterol and salmeterol are used twice daily, and indacaterol and olodaterol are used once daily. Arformoterol is the (R,R) enantiomer of formoterol, and is available for administration via a nebulizer. Other LABAs include vilanterol, which is available in combination formulations (e.g. fluticasone furoate/vilanterol) for once-daily use, and tulobuterol, which is available as a transdermal system (patch) in some countries.

The onset of action of formoterol and indacaterol is similar to that of salbutamol. Salmeterol, however, has a much slower onset of action, achieving bronchodilation within 15–30 minutes and a maximal effect within 2 hours. The maximal effect of olodaterol occurs after 1–2 hours.

Formoterol and salmeterol have been shown to significantly improve FEV_1, lung volumes and health-related quality of life, and reduce breathlessness and exacerbation rates and frequency. These LABAs have no effect on mortality or rate of decline of lung function.

Indacaterol significantly improves breathlessness, health status and exacerbation rate.

Anticholinergic agents affect cholinergic transmission, which is critical in maintaining normal airway smooth muscle tone.

M_1 muscarinic receptors mediate neural transmission in the vagal ganglia, and M_3 muscarinic receptors at the neuromuscular junctions mediate smooth muscle contraction (see Figure 7.1). Blockade of these receptors, particularly the M_3 receptors, can antagonize normal airway tone and thus result in bronchodilation. M_2 receptors have a feedback control function and may attenuate vagal activity.

Atropine has a modest bronchodilator effect, but is seldom used because of its other systemic effects. The anticholinergic agents most commonly used to achieve bronchodilation are quaternary amines (Table 7.4). When inhaled, these agents are absorbed very poorly, resulting in a high degree of local activity and a very low systemic side-effect profile.

Short-acting ipratropium bromide is most widely used. It has an onset of action slightly slower than salbutamol, demonstrating a bronchodilator effect in 10 minutes, a near-maximal effect in 30 minutes and a duration of action of 4–6 hours (see Figure 7.2). It is available in a metered-dose inhaler and as a nebulized solution. The approved dose in most countries (40 µg or 2 puffs every 6 hours) is probably not at the top of the dose–response curve.

TABLE 7.4

Amine anticholinergic bronchodilators

Drug	Inhaler (µg)	Nebulizer (mg)	Duration of action (hours)
Short-acting			
Ipratropium bromide	20–40 MDI	0.25–0.5	4–6
Oxitropium bromide	100 MDI	1.5	7–9
Long-acting			
Tiotropium	18 DPI, 5 SMI	–	24–36
Aclidinium bromide	322 DPI	–	12
Glycopyrronium bromide	44 (DPI)	–	24
Umeclidinium bromide	62.5*	–	24

*One inhalation once daily. DPI, dry-powder inhaler; MDI, metered-dose inhaler; SMI, soft mist inhaler.

As a result, improved bronchodilation and clinical effect can often be achieved with increased doses, and routine administration of 3 or 4 puffs has been suggested and is widely used. Interestingly, while the bronchodilator effect of ipratropium bromide is clearly shorter than that of salmeterol, both drugs result in a similar degree of improvement in exercise performance 6 hours after administration. This would be consistent with ipratropium bromide improving lung volumes and reducing dynamic hyperinflation over and above its ability to improve airflow.

Four long-acting anticholinergics have been approved: tiotropium bromide, glycopyrronium bromide and umeclidinium bromide are used once daily, and aclidinium bromide is used twice daily.

Tiotropium has been in use for the longest time. Its onset of action is slower than that of ipratropium bromide, but its duration of action is noticeably longer (see Figure 7.2). It reduces exacerbations and related hospitalizations, and improves symptoms and health status. It has also been shown to improve the effectiveness of pulmonary rehabilitation. In addition, tiotropium has been shown to prevent COPD exacerbations. Tiotropium has no effect on the rate of decline in lung function when added to other standard therapies.

The long-acting anticholinergics aclidinium and glycopyrronium have a similar action on lung function and breathlessness as tiotropium, but less information is available on the effects they have on other outcomes. Umeclidinium has demonstrated statistically significant improvement in lung function compared with tiotropium, and non-inferiority to glycopyrronium.

None of the long-acting anticholinergics has been assessed as treatment in acute settings. The side effects of anticholinergic agents in clinical use are generally mild and include dry mouth and a metallic taste. Closed-angle glaucoma may develop if drug is deposited in the eye. Men with prostate disease should be monitored for urinary tract effects, but these are uncommon. Aclidinium is rapidly hydrolyzed in the blood to inactive metabolites, which may reduce systemic exposure to anticholinergic effects. In patients with asthma, paradoxical bronchoconstriction with any inhaled medication can occur.

A post hoc meta-analysis raised questions about potential increased cardiovascular mortality in patients treated with anticholinergic agents.

However, a subsequent 4-year prospective trial of nearly 6000 patients comparing tiotropium with placebo found a decrease in cardiovascular events and a decrease in overall mortality that approached statistical significance in the tiotropium-treated group.

Theophylline is ineffective when administered topically as a bronchodilator and is usually used orally (Table 7.5), though it can be administered rectally. Intravenous formulations are no longer routinely used. Theophylline has several mechanisms of action, including inhibition of adenosine receptors and inhibition of multiple species of phosphodiesterase. The mechanism that leads to bronchodilatation is unclear. The traditional concept of phosphodiesterase inhibition leading to increases in cAMP and bronchodilatation has been called into question.

A number of theophylline preparations are available. Theophylline USP (*United States Pharmacopeia*) is comparatively inexpensive, but has a relatively short duration of action. It is cleaved by hepatic enzymes, which can be induced by a variety of stimuli; this leads to marked variations in theophylline clearance between patients and even in a given patient with changes in clinical state. Slow-release theophylline preparations for use once or twice daily provide steadier blood levels and are easier to use clinically. However, theophylline has major adverse side effects, which limit its use. These include CNS effects leading to nausea, vomiting and seizures, arrhythmias, relaxation of the lower gastroesophageal sphincter causing or worsening gastroesophageal reflux, diarrhea and headaches. Drug–drug interactions are common and further complicate use in clinical practice.

Many clinicians routinely check theophylline blood levels as toxic effects can be observed at levels only slightly above the traditional therapeutic range of 10–20 µg/mL. Recent practice, however, has been to

TABLE 7.5

Methylxanthines

Drug	Oral (mg)	Duration of action (hours)
Aminophylline	240	Variable up to 24
Theophylline (SR)	100–600	Variable up to 24

SR, slow release.

use theophylline at relatively low doses, maintaining blood levels in the 5–10 µg/mL range. This range is often associated with a satisfying clinical response and has an increased safety margin. A further reason for repeated testing is that, as noted above, theophylline is metabolized by the liver, and hepatic clearance can change, resulting in varying blood levels despite constant dosing and good compliance.

Theophylline can also be combined with β-agonist bronchodilators (with which cAMP levels may be raised synergistically), with anticholinergics and, as it does not meaningfully inhibit phosphodiesterase (PDE) 4, with roflumilast (see below).

Combination therapy. It is possible to combine bronchodilators from different classes. While some studies have suggested that a maximal bronchodilator effect can be achieved with a single agent given at sufficiently high dose, several large clinical trials have demonstrated an improvement in bronchodilator effect when a combination of β-agonist and anticholinergic bronchodilators are administered. A commercially available combination of salbutamol and ipratropium bromide (Combivent) has achieved widespread clinical acceptance. In general, combinations of β-agonist and anticholinergic bronchodilators are widely used. A number of fixed-dose combinations are in development and several have been approved (Table 7.6).

Non-bronchodilator effects of bronchodilators. It is likely that all drugs used to achieve bronchodilatation have a number of other effects. The clinical importance of these non-bronchodilator effects remains undefined.

LABAs and both long- and short-acting anticholinergic bronchodilators have been associated with a reduction in the frequency of COPD exacerbations. The mechanisms by which such an effect might be mediated are unclear. However, salmeterol has been demonstrated to directly affect airway epithelial cells in ways that may mitigate epithelial damage secondary to bacterial infection. β-agonists may inhibit the activity of inflammatory cells and act on blood vessels to reduce the formation of and accelerate the clearance of edema. Anticholinergic agents also have the potential for anti-inflammatory action by inhibiting the release of inflammatory mediators.

Theophylline may also have anti-inflammatory actions. It can improve diaphragmatic muscle contractility and may have other benefits, including

TABLE 7.6

β-agonist/anticholinergic combination therapy

Drug	Inhaler (µg)	Nebulizer (mg)	Duration of action (hours)
Short-acting β$_2$-agonist + anticholinergic			
Salbutamol/ ipratropium	100/20 SMI	–	6–8
Fenoterol/ ipratropium	200/80 MDI	1.25/0.5	6–8
Long-acting β$_2$-agonist + anticholinergic			
Indacaterol/ glycopyrronium	85/43 DPI	–	24
Vilanterol/ umeclidinium	25/62.5 DPI	–	24
Tiotropium/ olodaterol	2.5/2.5*	–	24

*Two inhalations once daily. DPI, dry-powder inhaler; MDI, metered-dose inhaler; SMI, soft mist inhaler.

a positive inotropic effect and a mild diuretic effect. In some studies, patients have reported subjective benefits from theophylline out of proportion to its modest bronchodilator activity.

The potential effects of bronchodilators on disease progression are discussed on pages 110–12.

Other pharmacological treatment options

Glucocorticosteroids. Oral corticosteroids should be avoided if at all possible in the management of stable COPD. Corticosteroid-induced side effects are relatively common and can be devastating in patients with COPD. Corticosteroid myopathy may further compromise individuals already relatively unable to exercise. Corticosteroid-induced osteoporosis may lead to fractures, which not only compromise mobility but also, if they occur in the spine or ribs, may lead to chest-wall splinting and an increased risk of pneumonia. Chronic administration of oral corticosteroids has been associated with increased mortality in patients with COPD. However, systemic corticosteroids may be of benefit during COPD exacerbations (Table 7.7). Treatment should be stopped after 7–14 days.

Inhaled corticosteroids improve airflow and symptoms. The mechanisms underlying this effect are unclear, but a reduction in airway edema has been suggested. It may take several weeks or even as long as 6 months for the benefits of this treatment to be observed. In general, the improvement in airflow, if there is any, is much less (averaging about 50 mL) than that achieved with bronchodilators (200–300 mL) (see above).

Inhaled corticosteroids also reduce the frequency and severity of exacerbations. This decrease appears to be associated with a beneficial effect on health status (quality of life), which is reasonable, as COPD exacerbations are associated with a worsening in health status. Several large studies have demonstrated a statistically significant benefit in terms of both exacerbations and health status. The effect on exacerbations is generally due to the effect in the most severely affected patients who experience the most frequent exacerbations, although milder cases may also benefit. Inhaled glucocorticosteroids should therefore be considered for patients with more severe airflow limitation ($FEV_1 < 60\%$ predicted) who experience frequent exacerbations, particularly if they are already receiving maximal bronchodilator therapy.

TABLE 7.7

Use of glucocorticosteroids in COPD

Systemic
- May be used for short-term treatment (7–14 days) during exacerbations
- Avoid chronic use
- No rationale for a therapeutic challenge

Inhaled
- Modest bronchodilator effect
- Reduce exacerbation frequency/severity
- Improve health status
- No effect on rate of decline in FEV_1

FEV_1, forced expiratory volume in 1 second.

Treatment with inhaled corticosteroids does not modify decline in FEV_1 or mortality in patients with COPD.

Adverse effects of inhaled corticosteroids are far fewer than those associated with systemic administration. Local side effects include thrush, dysphonia and oral candidiasis. Systemic effects, including skin fragility and bruising, are observed with some preparations. Adverse effects on bone density are controversial and have not been shown in most studies. Several meta-analyses have shown an association between inhaled corticosteroids and increased pneumonia risk. Agents that are cleared more rapidly from the circulation have fewer systemic side effects.

Corticosteroid/long-acting β-agonist inhaler combinations. Five combinations of a LABA and inhaled corticosteroid are currently available (Table 7.8): salmeterol–fluticasone proprionate (Seretide/Advair), formoterol–mometasone (Dulera), formoterol–beclometasone (Fostair) and formoterol–budesonide (Symbicort) are available for twice-daily use, and vilanterol–fluticasone furoate (Relvar/Breo) is available for once-daily use.

TABLE 7.8

Corticosteroid treatment options

Drug	Inhaler (µg)	Nebulizer (mg)
Inhaled corticosteroids		
Beclometasone*	50/400 MDI, DPI	0.04
Budesonide	100, 200, 400 DPI	0.2, 0.25, 0.5
Fluticasone	50–500 MDI, DPI	–
Combination long-acting β₂ agonists + corticosteroids		
Formoterol/Budesonide	4.5/160 MDI	9/320 DPI
Formoterol/Mometasone	10/200, 10/400 MDI	–
Salmeterol/ Fluticasone propionate	50/100, 200/250, 500 DPI	25/50, 125, 250 MDI
Vilanterol/ Fluticasone furoate	25/100 DPI	–
Formoterol/ Beclometasone*	6/100 MDI	–

*Beclomethasone in the USA. DPI, dry-powder inhaler; MDI, metered-dose inhaler.

The combination of an inhaled corticosteroid and a LABA is more effective than the individual components at improving lung function and health status and reducing exacerbations in patients with moderate to very severe COPD. These combinations have not been shown to produce a statistically significant effect on mortality. The increased risk of pneumonia has also been associated with combination therapy.

The addition of a LABA/inhaled corticosteroid combination to tiotropium has been shown to improve lung function and quality of life and may further reduce exacerbations.

Phosphodiesterase 4 inhibitors. Phosphodiesterases are a large family of enzymes that catalyze the degradation of cyclic nucleotides. PDE4 plays a particularly important role in inflammatory cells, which are thought to be important in COPD. As cAMP downregulates the activity of these cells and PDE4 degrades cAMP, PDE4 inhibitors were developed to treat COPD.

Roflumilast, 500 µg, taken once daily as an oral preparation, was the first of these agents to be approved for treatment of COPD. It reduces neutrophils in the sputum and results in modest (approximately 50 mL) improvements in airflow in all patients with COPD. Its primary benefit, however, is to reduce exacerbation risk in patients with chronic bronchitis. Roflumilast has been shown to reduce moderate-to-severe exacerbations in patients with chronic bronchitis and severe-to-very severe COPD with a history of exacerbations.

Adverse effects of roflumilast include nausea and diarrhea, both of which are usually mild and resolve with continued medication use over several weeks. The labeling in the USA contains a warning for mood changes and suicidality, as rare cases were observed in clinical trials. Roflumilast is metabolized in the liver and should not be used in subjects with liver failure (Child-Pugh class B or C). Weight loss can occur. This is usually self-limited and weight is regained when the medication is stopped. However, as patients with COPD who are underweight have a poorer prognosis, monitoring of weight should be routine with roflumilast use.

Vaccines. Influenza vaccination is recommended for all elderly patients since it can reduce mortality from influenza by around 50%. Vaccines that contain killed or live inactivated viruses are particularly recommended for elderly patients with COPD. The vaccine is adjusted each year to be effective against the appropriate strains of the virus, and the vaccination is usually given once a year in the autumn (or twice a year in the autumn and winter in some countries). Recent strategies have also advocated immunization of individuals likely to transmit influenza to patients with COPD.

Streptococcus pneumoniae is the most common cause of community-acquired pneumonia, and pneumococcal infection is more common in adults over the age of 50. Pneumococcal vaccination has been shown to be beneficial in reducing mortality from streptococcal pneumonia in an elderly population and, by extrapolation, might be expected to be effective in patients with COPD. While data regarding the specific use of pneumococcal vaccination in patients with COPD are limited, vaccination is recommended for those aged 65 or older and younger patients with COPD with significant comorbid conditions such as cardiac disease or severe airflow limitation ($FEV_1 < 40\%$ predicted).

α1-antitrypsin augmentation therapy may be appropriate for patients with severe hereditary α1-antitrypsin deficiency and established emphysema. The American Thoracic Society and European Respiratory Society recommend augmentation therapy for individuals with established airflow obstruction from α1-antitrypsin deficiency. The evidence of benefit is stronger in those with moderate FEV_1 impairment than those with severe obstruction. However, the therapy is expensive and is unavailable in many countries. Given the lack of demonstrable benefit in those without emphysema, augmentation therapy is not currently recommended in this population. Data from observational registries suggest that replacement therapy has benefits, but it is not recommended in patients with COPD that is unrelated to α1-antitrypsin deficiency.

Antibiotic therapy. Chronic use of several antibiotics has been tested to determine whether this type of therapy suppresses exacerbations in COPD. The best studied is azithromycin. In the MACRO study, azithromycin, 250 mg daily, was compared with placebo in 1142 subjects. Although the azithromycin group demonstrated a 27% reduction in exacerbation risk, there was an increase in resistant bacteria and a very modest decrease in hearing acuity. Subjects were carefully screened for potential cardiac problems, as azithromycin has been reported to increase arrhythmia risk.

Mucolytic agents (ambroxol, carbocisteine [carbocysteine], iodinated glycerol) have produced variable results in patients with COPD. Most studies have shown little or no change in lung function or symptoms. A systematic Cochrane collaborative review showed that mucolytic agents reduce episodes of acute-on-chronic bronchitis compared with placebo. Their use, however, remains controversial.

The mucolytic and antioxidant drugs N-acetylcysteine and carbocisteine have been shown to reduce the frequency of exacerbations of COPD in patients not taking inhaled corticosteroids.

Antitussives. Cough is a troublesome symptom in COPD, but it does have a protective role and therefore the use of antitussives is contraindicated in stable COPD.

Vasodilators. The rationale for the use of vasodilators is based on the relationship between pulmonary arterial pressure and mortality in COPD. Numerous vasodilators have been assessed. Most produce small changes in pulmonary arterial pressure, but at the expense of worsening ventilation–perfusion mismatching and therefore worsening gas exchange. There is therefore no indication for vasodilators in COPD.

Other drugs, such as leukotriene antagonists and nedocromil, have not been adequately assessed in COPD and cannot be recommended.

Modification of disease progression

The Lung Health Study was designed to determine whether inhaled ipratropium bromide could alter the rate of decline in lung function in patients with mild COPD. No effect was found, but the dose used (2 puffs three times daily) and relatively poor adherence could have compromised the results.

The TORCH (TOwards a Revolution in COPD Health) trial evaluated fluticasone, salmeterol, a combination of both drugs and placebo in a

3-year trial involving more than 6000 patients. The primary endpoint, mortality, did not achieve statistical significance, though a strong trend ($p=0.052$) was observed for the combination therapy compared with placebo (Figure 7.3a). Significant treatment benefits were a reduction in exacerbations, improvement in health status and a reduction in the rate of decline in lung function of 13–16 mL/year.

The UPLIFT (Understanding the Potential Long-term Impacts on Function with Tiotropium) trial also included nearly 6000 patients randomized to receive either tiotropium or placebo in addition to their usual care. Nearly 75% of patients were treated concurrently with an inhaled corticosteroid, a long-acting β-agonist or both. Tiotropium had no effect on the rate of decline in lung function for the groups as a whole. However, it was of significant benefit among those not treated with an inhaled corticosteroid or a long-acting β-agonist. Interestingly, the benefit of tiotropium was greater in those with moderate disease who had more rapid decline in lung function than in those with more severe disease. Importantly, tiotropium also had a significant effect in reducing exacerbations and a reduction in mortality was observed at the end of the treatment period (Figure 7.3b), although the mortality benefit lost statistical significance 30 days later, perhaps due to incomplete follow-up.

The reductions in exacerbations and improved health status clearly demonstrated in these two large clinical trials support the aggressive treatment of patients with COPD. A significant reduction in rate of decline in lung function is encouraging, though the clinical importance of this modest effect remains to be determined. Trends towards improved survival are also encouraging. Furthermore, while the results were not statistically significant, the strong trends observed allay safety concerns that have been raised with respect to bronchodilators and inhaled corticosteroids.

Assessing response to pharmacotherapy

Measurement of FEV_1 is not a reliable way of assessing response to treatment in patients with COPD. Simple questionnaires such as the COPD assessment test (CAT) may be useful in this respect, but directly questioning patients may be the most useful way to determine whether they have had a symptomatic response to treatment.

Figure 7.3 Effect of treatment on mortality in COPD. (a) The TORCH trial compared fluticasone, salmeterol, a combination of both drugs and placebo. A trend towards improved survival that did not reach statistical significance (p=0.052) was seen in the group receiving combination treatment compared with placebo. Reproduced from Celli BR et al. 2008, with permission of the American Thoracic Society © 2008. (b) The UPLIFT trial compared tiotropium with placebo in a group of patients with COPD, most of whom were treated with an inhaled glucocorticosteroid, a long-acting β-agonist or both. There was a statistically significant reduction in mortality in the tiotropium group at the end of treatment. Follow-up 30 days after discontinuation showed a trend toward improved survival that did not achieve significance (p=0.09). Reproduced from Tashkin DP et al. 2008, with permission from the Massachusetts Medical Society © 2008. All rights reserved.

- Has your treatment made any difference to you?
- Are you less breathless?
- Can you do things now that you could not do before?
- Can you do things now faster than before?
- Can you do the same things now but with less breathlessness?

Patient adherence to treatment is usually the most important determinant of whether a treatment will have benefit. Less than 50% of patients are fully adherent to therapeutic regimens for chronic diseases. Non-adherence may stem from poor understanding of treatment goals, difficulty in obtaining medications and, with inhaler medications, difficulty with or poor technique in using the device. Review of these issues, including patient demonstration of inhaler technique on a routine basis, is advisable.

Non-pharmacological treatment

Pulmonary rehabilitation. Previously, the main management goals in COPD were to prevent a deterioration of the condition, principally by encouraging smoking cessation, and to improve lung function and thus symptoms with bronchodilators. Substantial evidence now suggests that improving health status and functional ability is another attainable goal. The fact that the airflow limitation in COPD is largely irreversible means that the results of pharmacological therapy on lung function are, at best, modest. It is now known that, without changing airflow limitation, pulmonary rehabilitation can still improve both performance and health status.

There are no clear spirometric criteria to guide timing of referral for pulmonary rehabilitation. Referral should be considered for patients with persistent dyspnea, reduced exercise tolerance or impaired health status. Referral should not be delayed until lung disease has advanced to a point of significant limitations.

The principal goals of pulmonary rehabilitation are to reduce symptoms, improve health status, and increase physical and emotional participation in everyday activities. These goals are particularly relevant in the moderate-to-severe stages of COPD, when breathlessness may result in the avoidance of activity. This results in deconditioning of the skeletal muscles, which in turn leads to increasing disability, social isolation and

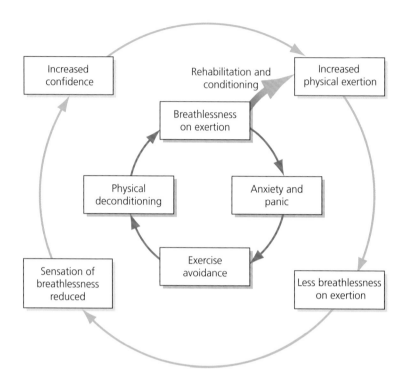

Figure 7.4 The vicious cycle of deconditioning and inactivity that occurs in COPD, and the effect of pulmonary rehabilitation.

depression. This compounds the problems of dyspnea and lack of fitness, and a vicious circle ensues, resulting in increasing dependence and disability and worsening quality of life (Figure 7.4).

The aim of pulmonary rehabilitation is to break this vicious circle of increasing inactivity, breathlessness and physical deconditioning, and improve exercise capacity and functional status.

The main components of a pulmonary rehabilitation program are:

* exercise training
* nutritional counseling
* education.

At all stages of COPD, patients appear to benefit from exercise training programs, which improve exercise tolerance and reduce symptoms of breathlessness and fatigue. Pulmonary rehabilitation has been assessed in numerous large clinical trials and the benefits are summarized in Table 7.9. Studies suggest that these benefits can be sustained after a single rehabilitation program if the patient maintains the exercise training at home.

The social isolation that accompanies severe COPD can lead to mood disturbances, which may require treatment. It is important to encourage social contact, and contact in the rehabilitation group may provide support. Generally, rehabilitation programs consist of two or three sessions per week for 6–10 weeks and provide a program of exercises that the patient also performs between sessions. The improvement seen with pulmonary rehabilitation programs seems to be long-lasting, persisting for at least a year. Follow-up is beneficial, and occasional repeat sessions have been offered in some centers that provide continuing support.

Rehabilitation involves a multidisciplinary group of healthcare professionals, and has been reported to have benefits in inpatient, outpatient and home settings. Selection criteria for pulmonary rehabilitation are still under investigation. Although benefits are seen in patients with a wide range of disability, those who are very severely disabled (e.g. those who are chair bound or have a modified Medical Research Council [mMRC] dyspnea score of 4 [see Table 3.2]) may not derive any benefit.

TABLE 7.9

Benefits of pulmonary rehabilitation in COPD

- Improves exercise capacity
- Reduces the perceived intensity of breathlessness
- Improves health-related quality of life
- Reduces the number of hospitalizations and length of hospital stay
- Strength and endurance training of the upper limbs improves arm function
- Benefits extend beyond the immediate period of training
- Improves survival
- Respiratory muscle training is beneficial, especially when combined with general exercise training
- Psychosocial intervention is helpful

It is important that motivated patients are selected for pulmonary rehabilitation. While many believe that inclusion of patients in a pulmonary rehabilitation program should be conditional on their participation in a smoking cessation program, there is no evidence that smokers will benefit less than non-smokers.

Exercise training to recondition skeletal muscles and improve exercise endurance is a key component of pulmonary rehabilitation. Bicycle ergometry and treadmill exercise are both suitable aerobic activities. A number of physiological variables, such as maximum oxygen consumption, maximum heart rate and maximum work performed are measured. A less complex approach utilizes a self-paced walking test (e.g. a 6-minute walking distance). Shuttle walking tests (see page 67) reflect an individual's peak oxygen consumption fairly accurately, provide more information than a 6-minute walking distance and are simpler to perform than a treadmill test.

Exercise training is performed regularly in a form that the patient will be able to continue at home during and after the rehabilitation program. The frequency of exercise varies from daily to weekly, the duration from 10 to 45 minutes and the intensity from 50% of peak oxygen consumption to maximum tolerated. Optimum training regimens have not been established, but maximal target exercise based on measured oxygen uptake has been reported to have superior results to programs based on predicted heart rate. Programs that include a regimen of varied intensities have also been reported to have superior results. The optimum length of a rehabilitation program has not been determined; suggestions from randomized controlled trials range from 6 to 10 weeks; however, the longer the program, the more beneficial the results.

Some programs include training of specific muscle groups, such as the upper limb girdle muscles, and aim to improve the patient's performance of specific tasks associated with daily living. There are no randomized controlled trial data to support the routine use of these exercises, but they may be useful in patients with comorbidity that restricts other forms of exercise and in those with severe COPD who find aerobic exercise too demanding.

The role of respiratory muscle training in pulmonary rehabilitation is still controversial. Training respiratory muscles for both strength and endurance has produced equivocal results in patients with COPD. However, inspiratory muscle training appears to have some additional benefit when undertaken as part of a comprehensive pulmonary rehabilitation program.

Nutritional counseling is based on the fact that the nutritional status of patients with COPD has an important effect on symptoms, disability and prognosis. Being overweight or underweight can be problematic. Around 25% of patients with moderate-to-severe COPD have a reduction in both their body mass index (BMI) and fat-free mass index. A low BMI has been shown to be an independent risk factor for mortality in patients with COPD (see Figure 2.4).

Management of underweight patients. The cause of malnutrition in COPD is complex and may relate to raised levels of various cytokines, including tumor necrosis factor. Breathlessness while eating can lead to reduced calorie intake and patients should be encouraged to take small frequent meals. Any problems with dentition should be corrected, and any comorbidity that might result in weight loss should be dealt with. Nutritional support in the form of increased calorie intake is best accompanied by exercise regimens that have an anabolic action. Underweight COPD patients whose nutritional state improves in response to therapy may also improve respiratory muscle strength and survival.

Management of obese patients with COPD. Obese patients are more likely to have greater impairment of activity and a greater degree of breathlessness than patients of normal weight. These patients should be encouraged to lose weight while taking regular exercise.

Education is included in most pulmonary rehabilitation programs, though its effect is unclear. Smoking cessation is a critical part of pulmonary rehabilitation and may be facilitated by advice and support from the physician (see Chapter 6). Advice should also be given on drug treatment and how to manage exacerbations.

Oxygen therapy. For individuals with resting hypoxemia (oxygen saturation < 88% or partial pressure of oxygen in arterial blood [PaO_2] < 7.3 kPa [55 mmHg]), long-term administration of oxygen therapy ($\geq$ 15 hours/day) has been shown to:

- improve survival
- prevent progression of pulmonary hypertension
- decrease polycythemia.

The UK MRC trial of oxygen, 15 hours/day, showed an increase in 5-year survival from 25% to 41% (compared with no oxygen). The Nocturnal Oxygen Therapy Trial (NOTT) showed that continuous oxygen therapy for a mean period of 17.7 hours/day was more beneficial in terms of survival than use for only 12 hours/day, which conferred no benefit. It is debatable whether oxygen therapy improves health status, but both mood and indices of depression improve.

Oxygen therapy reduces the oxygen costs of breathing and minute ventilation, thus reducing the sensation of breathlessness. It has been given to control severe breathlessness on exercise. Recent data suggest that ambulatory oxygen therapy improves the benefits obtained from exercise training programs.

When given during exercise, oxygen therapy increases walking distance by optimizing oxygen uptake and utilization by the muscles. However, there are no data to indicate whether long-term continuous oxygen therapy improves exercise capacity. Oxygen is administered during exercise to patients who usually fit the criteria for long-term oxygen therapy and to those who experience significant oxygen desaturation during exercise. A study evaluating the benefits of long-term oxygen for patients with COPD who are not hypoxic at rest but who desaturate with exercise is under way.

The goal of oxygen therapy is to increase PaO_2 to at least 8 kPa (60 mmHg) or to produce a percentage oxygen saturation of arterial blood (SaO_2) of at least 90% to ensure adequate oxygen delivery to vital organs.

Indications for long-term oxygen therapy in patients with COPD are:
- PaO_2 below 7.3 kPa (55 mmHg) or SaO_2 below 88%, with or without hypercapnia, confirmed on two occasions over a 3-week period
- PaO_2 between 7.3 and 8 kPa (55 and 60 mmHg) with evidence of pulmonary hypertension or peripheral edema, indicating cor pulmonale or polycythemia (hematocrit > 55%).

The need for oxygen therapy should be assessed when the patient is in a clinically stable state, at least 6 weeks after the last exacerbation and when other drug therapy has been optimized.

Delivery of long-term oxygen therapy is usually by an oxygen concentrator via nasal prongs at a flow rate of 2–3 liters/minute. Patients who desaturate during exercise are often told to increase the flow rate during exercise. Portable oxygen can also be provided by liquid oxygen and a portable device or by lightweight oxygen cylinders.

Ambulatory oxygen. A number of studies have shown that oxygen delivered during exercise can reduce the sensation of exercise-induced dyspnea and improve exercise tolerance. However, there is little evidence that the improvement seen in these laboratory studies is translated into improvements in exercise during daily living. In addition, compliance with ambulatory oxygen is poor. There is no good evidence that the use of short bursts of oxygen to relieve breathlessness before or after exercise is beneficial.

Oxygenation during air travel may be insufficient for patients with severe COPD who should, in any case, seek advice about any form of travel. Modern aircraft cabin pressures have oxygen levels equivalent to those 1500–2500 m (5000–8000 feet) above sea level; that is, an ambient oxygen pressure of 15–18 kPa (112–135 mmHg). This means that, in a healthy individual, the PaO_2 will decrease from 12 to 8.7 kPa (90 to 65 mmHg) and the SaO_2 from 96% to 90%. This reduction in oxygenation may be hazardous in a patient with severe lung disease and hypoxia unless supplementary oxygen is given during the flight. Patients with COPD are considered able to fly safely, with supplementary oxygen, if:

- FEV_1 is over 25% of the predicted value
- PaO_2 during the flight will be over 6.7 kPa (50 mmHg).

Patients with a resting PaO_2 at sea level of over 9.3 kPa (70 mmHg) may safely fly without supplementary oxygen.

If there is any doubt about the advisability of air travel, patients can be referred to a respiratory physician, who may perform a hypoxic challenge in which the patient breathes air with reduced levels of oxygen to assess their likely response to the levels of oxygen present during air travel.

Ventilatory support. The success of non-invasive intermittent positive-pressure ventilation (NIPPV) in patients with respiratory failure during exacerbations of COPD has led to its use in patients with chronic respiratory failure due to very severe COPD. Several studies have examined the use of ventilatory support in such patients but have found no convincing evidence that this treatment produces a long-term survival advantage over oxygen therapy alone. Given the conflicting evidence for the use of long-term NIPPV, it cannot be recommended for the routine treatment of patients with chronic respiratory failure due to COPD. However, a combination of NIPPV with long-term oxygen therapy may help some patients with severe daytime hypercapnia.

Surgical treatment

Bullectomy. Some patients with COPD develop large cyst-like spaces, or bullae, in the lungs, which tend to compress the more normal areas of the lung (see page 17). Removal of bullae that do not contribute to gas exchange may allow decompression of the adjacent lung parenchyma. Bullae can be detected on plain chest radiographs, but are better viewed on CT scans, which also permit the assessment of emphysema in the remaining lung (see Figure 5.2b). This may be an important determinant of the success of bullectomy.

A range of surgical procedures has been used, including bronchoscopic techniques using laser ablation. In carefully selected patients, such a procedure can improve lung function and symptoms of breathlessness. Patients who would benefit are those who have normal or minimally reduced diffusing capacity in the lung for carbon monoxide (DLco), and those who are not hypoxemic and who have good perfusion in the remaining lung, as assessed by lung perfusion scanning. Individuals less likely to benefit are those with pulmonary hypertension, hypercapnia and severe emphysema in the remaining non-bullous lung.

Lung volume reduction surgery removes emphysematous parts of the lung to decrease overinflation, thus improving the mechanical efficiency of the respiratory muscles, particularly the diaphragm. Lung volume reduction surgery also increases the elastic recoil pressure of the lung, so improving expiratory flow rates. This operation can be performed unilaterally or bilaterally using mediastinotomy or video-assisted thoracoscopy. Mortality in good centers is less than 5%. Bronchoscopic lung volume reduction surgery is also being performed to reduce emphysematous areas of the lung via insertion of endobronchial valves or coils that promote atelectasis of emphysematous lung.

Selection criteria for those who would derive most benefit are not fully established, although most studies select patients with an FEV_1 less than 35% of the predicted value, a PaO_2 less than 6 kPa (45 mmHg), predominant upper-lobe emphysema on the CT scan and a residual volume of more than 200% of the predicted value. Studies have shown that very severely affected patients with homogeneous disease and an FEV_1 or DLco less than 20% of the predicted value do not benefit; indeed, there is increased mortality in this group. Conversely, the US National Emphysema Treatment Trial identified individuals with upper-lobe disease and exercise limitation despite optimal medical treatment and rehabilitation as a group of good responders.

Lung volume reduction surgery has been shown to improve FEV_1, decrease total lung capacity, and improve exercise tolerance and quality of life; these effects may last for more than 2 years. In addition, longer-term follow-up has shown that lung volume reduction surgery leads to an improvement in maximal work capacity and health-related quality of life, a reduction in exacerbation frequency and improved survival. These beneficial effects are largely seen in those patients with predominant upper-zone emphysema and poor exercise tolerance. The efficacy of surgical and bronchoscopic lung volume reduction also depends on the presence of collateral ventilation to the diseased lobe (detected by the presence of an incomplete fissure between the lung lobes on CT scanning). Lung volume reduction surgery is expensive and should be reserved for carefully selected patients.

Lung transplantation. In patients with very advanced COPD, lung transplantation has been shown to improve health status and functional capacity, though it does not convey a survival benefit. The main criteria for lung transplantation are a Bode index (Body mass index, Obstruction, Dyspnea, Exercise; see Table 4.2) of 7–10 and one of the following:
- history of exacerbation associated with acute hypercapnia
- $PaCO_2$ over 6.7 kPa (50 mmHg)
- secondary pulmonary hypertension or cor pulmonale despite oxygen therapy
- FEV_1 less than 20% of the predicted value, with either DLco less than 20% predicted or homogeneous distribution of emphysema.

121

The number of lung transplants is limited by a shortage of donors. Complications after transplantation in patients with COPD include rejection, bronchiolitis obliterans and opportunistic infection. Bronchiolitis occurs in 30% of patients surviving for 5 years and may be fatal. Patients require long-term immunosuppressive therapy.

Palliative and end of life care

COPD may cause a gradual decline in health status and an increase in symptoms and exacerbations that result in increased risk of death. Latest projections estimate that COPD will become the fourth leading cause of death worldwide by 2030. Mortality following hospitalization for an acute exacerbation is between 25% and 80%. Deaths from respiratory failure, cardiovascular disease and malignancies are the primary cause of death in patients with COPD. Thus, palliative care/end of life care are important considerations in patients with advanced COPD. End of life care should be provided to patients with a life expectancy of less than 6 months. The goal of palliative care is to reduce suffering and give the best quality of life for patients and their families.

Physicians should bear in mind that not all patients will be ready for such a discussion the first time it is broached, but when they are, the main areas to cover are:

- likely disease course and prognosis
- advance healthcare directives
- symptom management
- psychosocial and spiritual concerns, with appropriate referral as required.

The course of COPD, particularly as the disease advances, is associated with episodes of acute increases in symptoms. These flare-ups or exacerbations can last from several days to weeks, and may occur several times a year with varying frequency in different individuals. These debilitating events result in unscheduled visits to healthcare professionals, hospitalizations and, occasionally, a need for ventilatory support and increased mortality.

Key points – therapy in stable disease

- Bronchodilators are the first-line treatment in COPD; they can be effectively used concurrently and also have beneficial non-bronchodilator effects.
- Inhaled glucocorticosteroids can improve airflow modestly and can reduce the frequency and severity of exacerbations.
- Short courses (7–14 days) of systemic corticosteroids may help following exacerbations, but should not be used over the long term.
- Optimum clinical benefits require an integrated program combining pulmonary rehabilitation with pharmacotherapy.
- Influenza vaccination is recommended for patients with COPD; there is also some evidence to support pneumococcal vaccination.
- Surgical removal of large bullae and lung volume reduction surgery may improve lung function and symptoms in carefully selected patients.
- Lung transplantation in patients with very advanced COPD improves health status and functional capacity, though it does not convey a survival benefit.
- Rehabilitation has been shown to be beneficial in terms of improving exercise tolerance, symptoms of breathlessness and fatigue in patients with COPD.

Key references

Calverley PM, Anderson JA, Celli B et al. Salmeterol and fluticasone propionate and survival in chronic obstructive pulmonary disease. N Engl J Med 2007;356:775–89.

Celli BR, MacNee W. Standards for the diagnosis and treatment of patients with COPD: a summary of the ATS/ERS position paper. Eur Respir J 2004;23:932–46.

Celli BR, Thomas NE, Andersen JA et al. Effect of pharmacotherapy on rate of decline of lung function in COPD: Results from the TORCH Study. Am J Respir Crit Care Med 2008;178:332–8.

Chapman KR, Burdon J, Piitulainen E et al. Augmentation therapy is disease modifying in alpha-1 antitrypsin deficiency. Interim analysis of the RAPID extension study. Am J Respir Crit Care Med 2014;189:A5788 [Abstract].

Furumoto A, Ohkusa Y, Chen M et al. Additive effect of pneumococcal vaccine and influenza vaccine on acute exacerbation in patients with chronic lung disease. *Vaccine* 2008;26:4284–9.

Global Initiative for Chronic Obstructive Lung Disease (GOLD). Pathogenesis, pathology, and pathophysiology. In: *Global Strategy for the Diagnosis, Management, and Prevention of COPD*. Updated December 2015. www.goldcopd.org, last accessed 19 January 2016.

Lacasse Y, Goldstein R, Lasserson TJ, Martin S. Pulmonary rehabilitation for chronic obstructive pulmonary disease. *Cochrane Database Syst Rev* 2006:CD003793.

Mitrouska R, Tzanakis N, Siafakas NM. Oxygen therapy in COPD. *Eur Resp Mon* 2006;38:302–12.

National Emphysema Treatment Trial Research Group. A randomized trial comparing lung-volume-reduction surgery with medical therapy for severe emphysema. *N Engl J Med* 2003;348:2058–73.

National Institute for Clinical Excellence (NICE). *Chronic Obstructive Pulmonary Disease: Management of COPD in adults in primary and secondary care*. www.nice.org.uk/guidance/cg101

Rennard SI. Anticholinergics in combination bronchodilator therapy in COPD. In: Spector SL, ed. *Anticholinergic Agents in the Upper and Lower Airways*. New York: Marcel Dekker, 1999:119–36.

Rennard S, Thomashow B, Crapo J et al. Introducing the COPD Foundation Guide for Diagnosis and Management of COPD, recommendations of the COPD Foundation. *COPD* 2013;10:378–89.

Russi EW, Imfeld S, Boehler A et al. Surgical treatment of chronic COPD. *Eur Resp Mon* 2006;38:359–74.

Schenkein JG, Nahm MH, Dransfield MT. Pneumococcal vaccination for patients with COPD: current practice and future directions. *Chest* 2008;133:767–74.

Siafakas NM, Celli BR. Overall management of stable COPD. In: *Management of Chronic Obstructive Pulmonary Disease. Eur Respir Mon* 2006;38:258–65.

Szafranski W, Cukier A, Ramirez A et al. Efficacy and safety of budesonide/formoterol in the management of chronic obstructive pulmonary disease. *Eur Respir J* 2003;21:74–81.

Tashkin DP, Celli B, Senn S et al. A 4-year trial of tiotropium in chronic obstructive pulmonary disease. *N Engl J Med* 2008;359:1543–54.

Tashkin DP, Rennard SI, Martin P et al. Efficacy and safety of budesonide and formoterol in one pressurized metered-dose inhaler in patients with moderate to very severe chronic obstructive pulmonary disease: results of a 6-month randomized clinical trial. *Drugs* 2008;68:1975–2000.

Troosters T, Donner CF, Schols AMWJ et al. Rehabilitation in COPD. *Eur Resp Mon* 2006;38:337–58.

8 Acute exacerbations

Acute exacerbations of chronic obstructive pulmonary disease (COPD), particularly those that result in hospitalization, place a large burden on healthcare resources. It has been estimated that, in an average UK Health Authority with a population of 250 000, there will be 14 200 consultations with a primary care physician and 680 hospital admissions for exacerbations of COPD each year. In the UK, respiratory admissions account for 25% of all acute emergency admissions, and COPD accounts for more than half of these, representing more than 200 000 hospital admissions per year. Recent studies have suggested that up to 50% of patients do not report exacerbations, so the true frequency is much higher than the number of consultations with primary care physicians suggests. Thus, the healthcare burden imposed by exacerbations of COPD is enormous. Annual costs in the USA are estimated at nearly $29.5 billion and $20.4 billion in direct and indirect costs, respectively. The comparable annual figure in the EU is €80 billion in total costs.

Since exacerbations increase in frequency and require a greater level of care as COPD progresses, most costs are incurred towards the end stage of the disease. General healthcare costs are also increased in patients with COPD, emphasizing the multisystem problems faced by this patient group.

Definition

There is no general agreement on the definition of an exacerbation of COPD. Most are based on increasing symptoms and/or increased healthcare utilization. A commonly used definition characterizes exacerbations based on the type and number of symptoms, such as increases in dyspnea, sputum volume or sputum purulence with or without symptoms of upper respiratory infection (Table 8.1). Fatigue may also be prominent.

The severity of an exacerbation can also be defined in terms of increasing healthcare utilization as: mild (self-managed by the patient at home); moderate (requiring treatment by the primary care physician and/ or hospital outpatient attendance); or severe (resulting in admission to

125

TABLE 8.1

Definition of COPD exacerbation

Type I

Three of: increased breathlessness, sputum volume or sputum purulence

Type II

Two of: increased breathlessness, sputum volume or sputum purulence

Type III

One of: increased breathlessness, sputum volume or sputum purulence

plus

one of the following symptoms:

- upper respiratory infection (sore throat, nasal discharge) within the past 5 days
- fever without other cause
- increased wheezing
- increased cough
- increase in respiratory or heart rate by 20% compared with baseline

Adapted from Anthonisen et al. 1987.

hospital). The severity of an exacerbation and the consequent healthcare utilization may depend on the severity of the underlying COPD.

Exacerbations of COPD are characterized by worsening pulmonary gas exchange and increasing hypoxemia (Table 8.2). Respiratory failure may develop in those patients with severe underlying disease or during severe exacerbations. Deterioration in gas exchange is largely due to an increased ventilation–perfusion mismatch. Hypoxemia during an exacerbation of COPD is usually due to increased areas of lung with low ventilation: perfusion ratios.

The hypercapnia of respiratory failure in some exacerbations is due to a number of factors including the increased work of breathing resulting from the increase in airways resistance and increase in systemic carbon dioxide production, and respiratory muscle fatigue. Sustained worsening is defined as symptoms worse than normal for at least 24 hours. A staging

TABLE 8.2

Physiological changes in COPD exacerbations

- Worsening hypoxemia primarily due to an increase in areas of the lungs with a low ventilation:perfusion ratio
- Increased dead space (wasted ventilation) as areas of the lung with a high ventilation:perfusion ratio increase
- Increased resistance to airflow in the upper and lower airways
- Increased work of breathing
- Hypercapnia in patients with underlying severe COPD or during severe exacerbation
- Pulmonary hypertension

TABLE 8.3

Staging of COPD exacerbations based on healthcare utilization

Severity	Level of healthcare utilization
Mild	Patients have an increased need for medication, which they can manage in their own normal environment
Moderate	Patients have an increased need for medication and feel the need to seek additional medical assistance
Severe	Patients/caregivers recognize obvious and/or rapid deterioration in condition, requiring hospitalization

system for exacerbations of COPD using clinical descriptors to characterize acute exacerbations has been proposed (Table 8.3).

Pathophysiology

Pathology studies of exacerbations in COPD have been performed on postmortem material and bronchial biopsies. Inflammation has also been assessed by non-invasive surrogate markers in sputum and breath. Relatively few of these last studies have involved patients with COPD, and patient numbers have been small.

It has been assumed that increased inflammation in the airways is a characteristic feature of exacerbations of COPD. However, the presence of increased inflammation, and particularly the type of inflammation, is controversial and depends on whether the inflammatory response is assessed in sputum, bronchoalveolar lavage fluid or bronchial biopsy, and on the severity of the exacerbation. The few studies of biopsies from patients with exacerbations of COPD have predominantly comprised patients with chronic bronchitis with mild airflow limitation; in some of these studies, increased levels of eosinophils were present in induced sputum and in bronchial biopsies from patients with exacerbations. However, neutrophils are also present in increased numbers in the bronchial walls and in bronchoalveolar lavage fluid in exacerbations of COPD.

Surrogate markers of inflammation, such as sputum levels of tumor necrosis factor α, interleukin (IL)-8 and IL-6, have been shown to be elevated in exacerbations of COPD. Oxidative stress is a major component of airway inflammation in COPD. Surrogate markers of oxidative stress are known to be elevated, compared with levels in healthy smokers, in the blood and exhaled breath of patients with stable COPD, and are further increased during exacerbations of COPD.

Etiology

The main etiologic factors in exacerbations of COPD are thought to be bacterial and viral infections, and air pollutants. Other factors associated with exacerbations of COPD are social deprivation and changes in temperature. However, in around 30% of exacerbations of COPD, no obvious etiologic factor is found.

Bacteria. Between 30% and 50% of patients with exacerbations of COPD have a positive sputum culture for bacteria. However, around 20–30% of clinically stable patients also have a positive bacterial culture from sputum. Bronchoscopic protected specimen brush biopsies show that bacteria are present in the lower airways in greater numbers during exacerbations than in the stable clinical state, suggesting infection. The main organisms present in sputum in exacerbations of COPD are *Haemophilus influenzae*, *Streptococcus pneumoniae* and *Moraxella catarrhalis*. Gram-negative bacteria, such as *Pseudomonas aeruginosa*, are less common during exacerbations of COPD, but occur with increasing frequency in patients with severe airflow limitation. In some studies, atypical bacterial pathogens such as *Chlamydia pneumoniae* have been found during exacerbations of COPD. Changes in bacterial strain have also been associated with acute exacerbations.

Respiratory viruses. Several studies have shown that viruses (mainly influenza and rhinovirus) are present in around 30% of acute exacerbations of COPD. They are associated with increased inflammation in the airways and a more prolonged time to the resolution of symptoms.

Air pollution is now a well-established cause of exacerbations of COPD. Epidemiological studies show links between the levels of particulate air pollution and emergency admissions for exacerbations of COPD. Other air pollutants, such as ozone, have also been associated with exacerbations of COPD in epidemiological studies.

Natural history
Studies in the 1960s, particularly in the UK, suggested that exacerbations of COPD were associated with small and transient decreases in respiratory function, and therefore did not alter the natural history of the disease. However, this view has since been challenged, and it is believed there may be a small but significant accelerated decline in lung function as a result of exacerbations of COPD. There are several large population studies showing that the number of exacerbations experienced increases with the severity of the underlying disease. The median number of exacerbations in patients with severe COPD is around 2.2–2.5 exacerbations per year. Frequent exacerbations (more than two per year) are associated with a poor quality of life, increased decline in pulmonary function and increased mortality. The frequency of exacerbations can be accurately assessed by patient recall.

Follow-up of patients with exacerbations of COPD shows a high readmission rate of around 30% over the first 3 months. Patients with recurrent exacerbations (three or more exacerbations per year) have a higher mortality rate and a decreased quality of life.

Symptoms and signs

Patients with acute exacerbations typically present with increased cough, changes in sputum volume and/or purulence, and increased breathlessness, wheezing and chest tightness. The clinical history, examination and arterial blood gases are used to assess the severity of the exacerbation in order to judge whether a patient requires admission to hospital. A number of other non-specific symptoms, such as malaise, sleepiness, fatigue and confusion, may occur in exacerbations. Fever may be present and an increase in sputum purulence suggests a bacterial cause, as does a history of chronic sputum production. The severity of the exacerbation is assessed from the medical history, particularly the severity of the underlying COPD, the presence of pre-existing comorbidities, the physical examination and gas measurements (Table 8.4).

Respiratory failure may or may not be present, as may cyanosis and the flapping tremor of hypercapnia, but these signs are rather insensitive. Pulse oximetry can rapidly provide information about oxygen saturation, but arterial blood gases should be measured in all patients with severe

TABLE 8.4

Assessment of severity of COPD exacerbations

History

- Severity of underlying airflow limitation is measured by forced expiratory volume in 1 second
- Duration or severity of new symptoms
- Number of previous episodes (exacerbations/hospitalizations)
- Comorbidities
- Current treatment regimen

Signs of severity

- Use of accessory muscles of respiration
- Worsening or new onset of cyanosis
- Hypercapnia
- Development of peripheral edema
- Reduced alertness

exacerbations. Peak expiratory flow measurements are not as useful for determining the need for hospital admission in COPD as they are in asthma. Chest radiographs may be useful to diagnose conditions that may mimic symptoms of an exacerbation (see below and page 133).

The presence of purulent sputum during an exacerbation is usually a sufficient indication for starting empirical antibiotic treatment. If an exacerbation does not respond to such treatment, sputum should be cultured and bacterial sensitivities identified.

Several conditions may mimic COPD exacerbations including congestive cardiac failure, pneumothorax, pneumonia, pulmonary embolism and cardiac arrhythmia. It is particularly important to consider these differential diagnoses in patients with exacerbations of COPD who do not respond to treatment.

Prevention

Prevention or reduction in the severity or length of exacerbations of COPD is a major goal of management. Influenza vaccination is recommended since it reduces hospitalization for pneumonia in elderly patients with COPD during epidemics. Vaccination against streptococcal pneumonia is available and is effective in preventing the complications of the infection.

There is now evidence that a range of drugs including long-acting β-agonists (LABAs), inhaled corticosteroids and long-acting anticholinergic agents can reduce the frequency of exacerbations. The combination of a LABA and an inhaled corticosteroid is more effective in reducing exacerbations than either agent individually.

The use of mucolytic agents in COPD has been evaluated in a number of studies. The effects on the frequency of exacerbations have been mixed. There is, however, some evidence that, in patients with COPD who have not been treated with an inhaled corticosteroid, mucolytics may reduce exacerbations.

Management

The aims of management in exacerbations of COPD are to relieve airway obstruction, correct hypoxemia, address any comorbid disorder that may contribute to respiratory deterioration and treat any precipitating causes such as infection.

Management at home. Most exacerbations of COPD are treated in primary care; only a minority of patients are admitted to hospital.

Bronchodilators. The dose and the frequency of use of bronchodilators are increased in home management of exacerbations of COPD. If not already used, therapy with multiple bronchodilator classes may be added if symptoms are not improving. In the most severe cases, high-dose nebulized bronchodilators can be given on a regular or as-required basis for several days. However, there is evidence that the use of multiple doses of bronchodilators by metered-dose inhaler with a spacer device has an effect similar to that of nebulized bronchodilators in exacerbations of COPD. When a nebulizer is used, it is probably safer to use air as the driving gas, rather than oxygen, and to continue oxygen therapy via nasal prongs. The long-term use of nebulized therapy after acute exacerbations of COPD is not routinely recommended.

Antibiotics. The use of antibiotics in exacerbations of COPD is still controversial. In mild-to-moderate exacerbations, sputum culture is not usually necessary. Patients with purulent sputum and at least one of increased breathlessness or increased sputum production show greater improvement with antibiotics than with placebo during exacerbations of COPD. Simple antibiotics, modified according to local bacterial resistance patterns, should be used. Amoxicillin can be given in most cases as first-line treatment, or co-amoxiclav in those who fail to respond or who are known or suspected to have β-lactamase-producing organisms in their sputum. Clarithromycin or doxycycline is an alternative in patients who are hypersensitive to penicillins.

Glucocorticosteroids. The use of corticosteroids in exacerbations of COPD is now well established. Several controlled trials have shown that systemic corticosteroids achieve a greater improvement in spirometry, shorten recovery time, reduce length of stay in hospital, reduce the risk of early relapse and have fewer treatment failures than placebo. The exact dose of corticosteroids that should be given has not yet been established, but present evidence suggests that 40 mg/day for 5 days is appropriate.

Hospital treatment. Provisional guidelines provide indications for hospital admission for acute exacerbations of COPD (Table 8.5).

TABLE 8.5

Indications for hospital admission for acute exacerbations of COPD

The more referral indicators that are present, the more likely the need for admission to hospital

	Treat at home	Treat in hospital
Ability to cope at home	Yes	No
Breathlessness	Mild	Severe
General condition	Good	Poor and deteriorating
Level of activity	Good	Poor or confined to bed
Cyanosis	No	Yes
Worsening peripheral edema	No	Yes
Level of consciousness	Normal	Impaired
Already receiving long-term oxygen therapy	No	Yes
Social circumstances	Good	Living alone or not coping
Acute confusion	No	Yes
Rapid rate of onset	No	Yes
Changes on the chest radiograph	No	Present
Arterial pH level	≥ 7.35	< 7.35
PaO_2	≥ 7 kPa (52 mmHg)	< 7 kPa (52 mmHg)

PaO_2, partial pressure of oxygen in arterial blood.
Source: British Thoracic Society Guidelines for the management of chronic obstructive pulmonary disease. *Thorax* 1997;52(suppl 5):S1–S28.

Blood gases should be measured in all severe exacerbations of COPD. A partial pressure of oxygen in arterial blood (PaO_2) below 6.7 kPa (50 mmHg), a partial pressure of carbon dioxide in arterial blood ($PaCO_2$) above 9.3 kPa (70 mmHg) or a pH below 7.3 suggests a life-threatening episode that needs close monitoring or management in an intensive care unit (ICU).

The presence of a pulmonary embolism, which can mimic an exacerbation of COPD, can be very difficult to diagnose, particularly in patients with COPD. Chest radiographs are useful in diagnosis. A low diastolic blood pressure and an inability to increase the PaO_2 to more than 8 kPa (60 mmHg) despite oxygen therapy also suggest pulmonary embolism. Spiral computed tomography pulmonary angiography is the best tool available for diagnosis of pulmonary embolism. Ventilation/perfusion scanning is of no value in patients with COPD.

The first actions when treating patients hospitalized with an exacerbation of COPD are to provide controlled oxygen therapy and to determine whether the exacerbation is life-threatening, in which case admission to an ICU is indicated. Management of other acute exacerbations of COPD is summarized in Table 8.6.

Oxygen therapy aims to maintain adequate oxygenation (PaO_2 > 8 kPa [60 mmHg] or percentage oxygen saturation of arterial blood [SaO_2] of 88–92%) without worsening the hypercapnia. Many patients who have chronic hypoxemia will tolerate a lower PaO_2 (> 6.7 kPa [50 mmHg]) after administration of oxygen. Oxygen is given in inspired concentrations of 24–28% by Venturi mask or 1–2 liters/minute by nasal prongs. Arterial blood gases should be remeasured after 30–60 minutes to ensure satisfactory oxygenation without additional retention of carbon dioxide and consequent acidosis. Oxygen masks provide a more accurate inspired oxygen concentration, but nasal prongs are better tolerated.

Bronchodilator therapy can mitigate the effects of increased airway obstruction, namely increased respiratory work of breathing (hyperinflation, respiratory muscle mechanical disadvantage and impaired ventilation/perfusion matching), causing hypoxemia in patients with exacerbations of COPD. Short-acting β-agonists (SABAs) are preferred as initial bronchodilators in acute exacerbations. Although they are usually given in nebulized form, there is evidence that administration of β-agonists via metered-dose inhaler and spacer device is equally efficacious.

Nebulizers should be powered by compressed air rather than oxygen if the $PaCO_2$ is raised, to prevent worsening hypercapnia and acidosis. Oxygen administration via nasal prongs can continue at 1–2 liters/minute during nebulization.

TABLE 8.6

Management of severe but not life-threatening exacerbations of COPD

- Assess severity of symptoms, blood gases and chest radiograph
- Administer controlled oxygen therapy – repeat arterial blood gas measurement after 30 minutes
- Bronchodilators
  - increase dose or frequency
  - combine β-agonists and anticholinergic agents
  - use spacers or air-driven nebulizers
  - consider adding intravenous aminophylline, if needed
- Corticosteroids, oral or intravenous
- Antibiotics when signs of bacterial infection are present, given orally or occasionally intravenously
- Consider mechanical ventilation
- At all times:
  - monitor fluid balance and nutrition
  - consider subcutaneous heparin
  - identify and treat associated conditions (e.g. heart failure, arrhythmias)
  - closely monitor condition of the patient

If the response to a β-agonist is not prompt, or if the patient has a very severe exacerbation, the anticholinergic drug ipratropium bromide can be added.

The role of intravenous aminophylline in the treatment of COPD exacerbations is controversial. Studies have shown minor improvements in lung volumes following administration of aminophylline, but also worsening gas exchange. Monitoring of serum theophylline levels is recommended to avoid the side effects of these drugs.

Glucocorticosteroids have been shown to reduce symptoms and improve lung function effectively in patients with acute exacerbations of COPD. Currently, systemic corticosteroid, 40 mg/day for 5 days, is

135

recommended for all patients with an acute exacerbation in the absence of significant contraindications. Oral corticosteroids are preferable. Nebulized budesonide is an alternative to oral corticosteroid treatment in exacerbations without respiratory failure and is associated with a reduction in complications, such as hyperglycemia. Corticosteroids should be discontinued after the acute episode; clinical improvement with corticosteroids during the exacerbation does not indicate the need for long-term treatment with oral or inhaled corticosteroids.

Antibiotic therapy in exacerbations of COPD was the subject of a meta-analysis of nine randomized placebo-controlled trials. This analysis established a small but significant benefit, which was most evident in patients with the most symptoms. When two of the three cardinal symptoms (increasing breathlessness, increasing sputum volume and increasing sputum purulence) were present, with one of these being increased sputum purulence, there was a significant improvement following treatment with antibiotics compared with placebo.

In most cases, sputum Gram-stain or culture is unnecessary. Oral rather than intravenous antibiotics should be given. Failure to respond to simple antibiotics (as described above), the known presence of β-lactamase-producing organisms in sputum or severe exacerbations are all indications for a broader spectrum antibiotic, such as co-amoxiclav, a second- or third-generation cephalosporin or fluoroquinolone, or a newer macrolide.

Sputum clearance. Airway inflammation in exacerbations of COPD promotes mucus hypersecretion. There are no convincing data to support the use of pharmacological agents to improve mucokinetics during exacerbations. The use of mechanical techniques such as physiotherapy have no proven value in acute exacerbations, unless a large amount of sputum (> 25 mL) is produced daily or there is mucus plugging with lobar atelectasis. Physiotherapy is not recommended in patients with acute-on-chronic respiratory failure.

Diuretics are indicated in the presence of edema and raised jugular venous pressure.

Anticoagulants, specifically prophylactic subcutaneous heparin, should be administered to patients with severe exacerbations, particularly those who are immobile and those with acute-on-chronic respiratory failure.

Ventilatory support

The objectives of mechanical ventilatory support in patients with exacerbations of COPD are to reduce mortality and morbidity, and relieve symptoms. Ventilatory support includes both non-invasive ventilation using negative or positive pressure devices and invasive mechanical ventilation by endotracheal intubation.

Non-invasive intermittent ventilation has been shown in several randomized control trials in acute respiratory failure in COPD to reduce respiratory acidosis, the severity of breathlessness, the length of stay in hospital, the need for intubation and mortality. However, non-invasive ventilation is not appropriate for all patients (Table 8.7).

TABLE 8.7

Indications and contraindications for non-invasive ventilation

Indications

- Severe breathlessness; clinical signs suggestive of respiratory muscle fatigue such as use of accessory muscles and paradoxical abdominal motion
- Moderate-to-severe acidosis (pH ≤ 7.35) and/or $PaCO_2 > 6$ kPa (45 mmHg)
- Respiratory frequency > 25 breaths/minute

Exclusion criteria

- Respiratory arrest
- Cardiovascular instability (arrhythmias, hypotension, myocardial infarction)
- Change in mental status, uncooperative patient
- High aspiration risk
- Viscous or copious secretions
- Craniofacial trauma
- Nasopharyngeal abnormalities
- Extreme obesity

$PaCO_2$, partial pressure of carbon dioxide in arterial blood.

TABLE 8.8

Indications for invasive mechanical ventilation

- Unable to tolerate or failure of non-invasive ventilation
- Severe breathlessness or respiration rate > 35 breaths/minute
- Life-threatening hypoxemia
- Severe acidosis (pH < 7.25)
- Respiratory arrest
- Impaired mental status
- Vascular complications (hypotension)
- Other complications (metabolic, sepsis, pneumonia, pulmonary embolism)

Invasive mechanical ventilation. The indications for initiating invasive mechanical ventilation during exacerbations of COPD are shown in Table 8.8. Use of invasive ventilation in patients with end-stage COPD is influenced by the patient's wishes and the likelihood of reversing the precipitating events. A clear statement of the patient's own treatment wishes – an advance directive – may make these decisions easier.

Hospital discharge and follow-up

There are no data indicating the optimal duration of hospitalization for acute exacerbations of COPD, but suggested discharge criteria are listed in Table 8.9. Follow-up assessment 4–6 weeks after discharge from hospital is recommended (Table 8.10). To ensure that any abnormalities seen on chest radiograph have completely resolved, another radiograph should be taken at 6 weeks' follow up. Recommendations for re-imaging nodules incidentally detected on CT scan should be based on smoking history.

The presence of hypoxemia during an exacerbation of COPD should prompt rechecking of blood gases at discharge. If the patient remains hypoxemic, the need for long-term outpatient oxygen therapy should be assessed when the patient attains a stable state.

Randomized controlled trials have shown that 20–30% of patients hospitalized with acute exacerbations of COPD can be safely allowed home with support without adverse consequences.

TABLE 8.9

Discharge criteria for patients with acute exacerbations of COPD

- Inhaled β-agonist therapy is required no more frequently than every 4 hours
- Patient, if previously ambulatory, is able to walk across room
- Patient is able to eat and sleep without frequent disruption by dyspnea
- Patient has been clinically stable for 12–24 hours
- Arterial blood gases have been stable for 12–24 hours
- Patient (or home caregiver) fully understands correct use of medications
- Follow-up and home-care arrangements have been completed (e.g. visiting nurse, oxygen delivery, meal provision)
- Patient, family and physician are confident that patient can manage successfully

Key points – acute exacerbations of COPD

- Acute exacerbations of COPD are common and place a huge burden on healthcare resources.
- The main etiologic factors in acute exacerbations are bacterial infection, respiratory viruses and air pollution.
- Treatment includes oxygen, increased use of bronchodilators, antibiotics and short-term oral glucocorticosteroids.
- Exacerbations can be prevented by inhaled corticosteroids and vaccination against influenza.
- Most exacerbations of COPD are managed at home, but those with suspected respiratory failure should be admitted to hospital.
- Non-invasive ventilation has been shown to reduce mortality in patients with acute-on-chronic respiratory failure.

TABLE 8.10

Follow-up assessment for acute exacerbations of COPD 4–6 weeks after hospital discharge

- Assess ability to cope in usual environment
- Measure forced expiratory volume in 1 second
- Reassess inhaler technique
- Check patient's understanding of recommended treatment regimen
- Assess need for long-term oxygen therapy and/or home nebulizer (for patients with severe COPD)

Key references

Anthonisen NR, Manfreda J, Warren CPW et al. Antibiotic therapy in exacerbations of chronic obstructive pulmonary disease. *Ann Intern Med* 1987;106:196–204.

Davies L, Angus RM, Calverley PMA. Oral corticosteroid in patients admitted to hospital with exacerbations of COPD: a prospective randomized trial. *Lancet* 1999;354:456–60.

MacNee W. Acute exacerbations of COPD. Consensus conference on management of chronic obstructive pulmonary disease. *J R Coll Phys Edinb* 2002;32:1–46.

Niewoehner DE, Erbland ML, Deupree RH et al. Effect of systemic glucocorticoids on exacerbations of COPD. *N Engl J Med* 1999;340:1941–7.

Rodriguez-Roisin R. Towards a consensus definition for COPD exacerbations. *Chest* 2000;117:398S–401S.

Saint S, Bent S, Vittinghoff E, Grady D. Antibiotics in chronic obstructive pulmonary disease exacerbations. A meta-analysis. *JAMA* 1995;273:957–60.

Seemungal TAR, Donaldson GC, Bhowmik A et al. Time course and recovery of exacerbations in patients with COPD. *Am J Respir Crit Care Med* 2000;161:1608–13.

Seemungal TAR, Donaldson GC, Paul EA et al. Effect of exacerbation on quality of life in patients with COPD. *Am J Respir Crit Care Med* 1998;157:1418–22.

Siafakas NM, Vedzicha JA. Management of acute exacerbation of COPD. *Eur Respir Mon* 2006;38:387–400.

New therapies in development

Research in the area of COPD is vigorous, and current investigations are shedding new light on its pathogenesis. Advances in our understanding of the mechanisms responsible for the lung damage and the systemic aspects of COPD will enable new therapeutic targets to be identified (Table 9.1). Because of the high prevalence and burden of COPD, there is a correspondingly large potential market. The pharmaceutical industry has responded with major investments in exploring novel therapeutic targets, and a number of new agents are under investigation.

Improved understanding of disease

Recent improvements in our understanding of COPD are likely to lead to more sophisticated diagnostic and therapeutic approaches. Recognition that dyspnea is an inspiratory event and that dynamic changes related to respiratory rate are major contributors is likely to lead to improved physiological assessment of the COPD patient. Improvements in imaging technology, including high-resolution CT scanning and hyperpolarized gas MRI, hold great promise for better defining the anatomy of the lung of the COPD patient. These new technologies may help with patient selection for regional treatments; CT scanning is now mandatory before lung-volume reduction surgery.

Multiple dimensional assessments that incorporate physiology together with performance measures, symptom scores and other domains have proved highly useful in clinical trials. Investigation of similar measures in clinical practice is now under way. Improved methods to evaluate exacerbation frequency, severity and duration will improve both clinical trials and clinical management.

Improved methods of diagnosis

Fundamental changes in the way COPD is approached are also likely to change clinical practice. To date, COPD has been defined simply, and a diverse group of patients with a heterogeneous collection of conditions has

TABLE 9.1

Targets for novel therapies for COPD

Pro-inflammatory signaling
- Cytokines
- Cytokine receptors
- Cytokine receptor signaling pathway components

Inflammatory mediators
- Proteinases
  - serine
  - metalloproteinases
  - cysteine
- Oxidants
- Defensins
- Complement
- Injury pathways
  - apoptosis
  - cell adhesion factors

Neural pathways
- Modulator pathways
- Transmitters
- Receptor agonists/antagonists

Repair
- Growth factors
- Differentiation factors
- Stem cells

been grouped together. Treatments at present are symptom-based and attack common mechanisms shared by most patients. It is probable that, in the near future, more sophisticated diagnostic methods will be applied to identify subsets of patients who respond to more mechanistically based treatments. Such treatments may be much more effective than current therapies, albeit for a smaller proportion of patients. It may be that COPD will become fragmented into many conditions, each of which may include only a small group of patients. This approach holds particular promise for modifying the progressive nature of the disease.

Biomarkers. There is considerable interest in developing biomarkers as diagnostics for COPD. A biomarker is not needed to diagnose the presence of COPD, which is readily done with spirometry. Conversely, exacerbations are diagnosed clinically and a reliable biomarker could help guide therapy just as procalitonin and brain naturetic peptide have done for pneumonia and heart failure, respectively.

Biomarkers that reflect disease activity would greatly facilitate the development of novel treatments designed to alter the natural history of the disease. In addition, biomarkers may be able to identify patients who are at greater risk of exacerbation, hospitalization or death. Several have been proposed, but none has yet achieved widespread clinical use.

Potential for lung repair

Strikingly, studies have demonstrated that the lung has considerable capacity to repair itself following injury. In animal models, emphysema can be reversed by the administration of all-*trans*-retinoic acid. Similar studies are under way in humans to evaluate the use of agents selective for the retinoic acid receptor. Clinical trials with mesenchymal stem cells, which may have both anti-inflammatory effects as well as the potential to mediate repair, are also in progress. The possibility that lung function can be restored in patients with COPD is particularly exciting.

Prevention of COPD

The most important future direction, however, is prevention of COPD. Recognizing the risk factors for COPD, particularly cigarette smoking, makes this eminently feasible. Advances in preventing people from starting to smoke and in promoting cessation among established smokers could not only slow the progression of existing COPD, but also prevent new cases developing. Recent data from the USA demonstrated a decrease in mild airflow limitation among younger Americans in conjunction with a reduction in smoking initiation and prevalence, which may herald a downward slope of the COPD epidemic.

Useful resources

UK
Association of Respiratory Nurse Specialists
Tel: +44 (0)7740 117 902
info@arns.co.uk
www.arns.co.uk

Breathing Matters
Tel: +44 (0)20 3549 5979
www.breathingmatters.co.uk

British Lung Foundation
Helpline: 03000 030 555
helpline@blf.org.uk
www.blf.org.uk

British Thoracic Society
Tel: +44 (0)20 7831 8778
bts@brit-thoracic.org.uk
www.brit-thoracic.org.uk

USA
American Association for Respiratory Care
Tel: +1 972 243 2272
info@aarc.org
www.aarc.org

American College of Chest Physicians
Tel: +1 224 521 9800
Toll-free: 1 800 343 2227
www.chestnet.org

American Lung Association
Helpline: 1 800 548 8252
info@lung.org
www.lung.org

American Thoracic Society
Tel: +1 212 315 8600
ATSInfo@Thoracic.org
www.thoracic.org

COPD Foundation
Info line: +1 866 316 2673
info@COPDfoundation.org
www.COPDfoundation.org
Educational materials at
www.COPDfoundation.org/
Learn-More/Educational-Materials/
Downloads-Library.aspx

QUITNET
www.quitnet.com

Respiratory Nursing Society
www.respiratorynursingsociety.org

International
Action on Smoking and Health
www.ash.org.uk (UK)
Tel: +44 (0)207 404 0242
enquiries@ash.org.uk
www.ash.org (USA)
Tel: +1 202 659 4310
info@ash.org

COPD Association (Singapore)
info@copdas.com
www.copdas.com

European Respiratory Society
Tel: +41 (0)21 213 0101
www.ersnet.org

Global Initiative for Chronic
Obstructive Lung Disease
www.goldcopd.org

International Primary Care
Respiratory Group
Tel: +44 (0)1224 743753
BusinessManager@theipcrg.org
www.theipcrg.org

South Africa Thoracic Society
Tel: +27 21 650 3050
sarj@iafrica.com
www.pulmonology.co.za

The Lung Association (Canada)
Tel: +1 613 569 6411
Toll-free: 1 888 566 5864
www.lung.ca

The Thoracic Society of Australia
and New Zealand
Tel: +61 (0)2 9222 6200
info@thoracic.org.au
www.thoracic.org.au

FastTest

You've read the book ... now test yourself with key questions from the authors

- Go to the FastTest for this title
  FREE at fastfacts.com
- Approximate time **10 minutes**
- For best retention of the key issues, try taking the FastTest before and after reading

145

Index

BMA LIBRARY BRITISH MEDICAL ASSOCIATION